Prevent Tooth Decay and Gum Disease

How To Save Your Teeth and Your Health

Copyright © 2012 by Alicia J. Smith

All Rights Reserved

Image: FreeDigitalPhotos.net

Table Of Contents

Disclaimer	5
Introduction	6
The Connection Between Tooth Decay And Degenerative Disease	11
Why Your Teeth Decay	14
The Fluid Transport System Inside Your Teeth	18
Playing PH Roulette	24
Sources of Acid Erosion	27
Acid and Your Teeth	27
Acidic Foods and Beverages	29
Destroying Your Teeth One Sip and One Bite At A Time	30
Acid Reflux and Your Teeth	34
Vomiting And Your Teeth	35
Mature Dental Plaque Biofilm	36
Acidic Teeth Whitening Products	38
Diet and Dental Health	39
The Importance of Diet and Saliva	42
Calcitriol - Vitamin D3 and Diet	42

Diet, Physical Health and Dental Health	43
Customizing Your Diet	46
Thirteen Ways To Destroy Your Teeth	50
How Dental Procedures Impact Your Teeth and Your Health	53
Fillings	55
Crowns	58
Root Canals	62
Caring For Your Teeth	66
Treating Bleeding Gums and Aching Teeth	68
Temporary Tooth Repair	72
Cleaning and Sanitizing Your Teeth	74
Plaque Removal and Scaling	78
Brushing and Flossing	83
Dental Irrigation	89
Disinfecting Rinse	94
The Fluoride Controversy	97
Preventative Measures	107
The Golden Key To Success	111
Summary and Conclusion	115

Disclaimer

This book is offered solely for your information, education, and amusement. The author is merely a layman, not an expert in dental care, and you should interpret the author's opinions accordingly.

The information contained herein may, or may not be beneficial, and no claims are made to treat, cure, prevent, or diagnose any diseases. No health claims are intended, implied, made or offered. No medical advice, diagnosis, prevention, prescription, or cure is claimed or offered in this book.

The opinions set forth in this book are solely the opinions of the author and should not be taken as a substitute for seeking legitimate medical advice from your dentist or other medical provider.

The dental care information listed in this book has not been approved or endorsed by the FDA, AMA, NDA, or any other United States, State, County, City, or other agency.

Introduction

Thank you for choosing to read this book. You will benefit the most if you take the time to read each chapter in order. Skipping ahead to other chapters will leave you without the foundational knowledge you need to make accurate and informed decisions that can have long-term profound dental and overall health consequences.

It is one thing for someone to tell you that you should do something just because it is good for you. On the other hand, understanding the underlying reasons for taking specific actions will give you a concrete basis on which to make and keep your commitment to positive changes that can improve your dental and physical health.

Much of what you think you know about dental care and the cause of tooth decay are only half true. Although bacteria do play a role in tooth decay, they are not the primary driving factor. At any given time there are hundreds of different species of bacteria living in your mouth with a population numbering in the billions. If bacteria were the main cause of tooth decay, no one would have teeth left by the age of twenty because the bacteria would have already consumed them.

Are you aware that your body is designed to repair and

renew your teeth? A constant process is at work in your mouth that either maintains good dental health, or destroys it. One process removes the minerals from your tooth enamel; the other process builds minerals back up on your tooth enamel. This cycle is called demineralization and remineralization, and when the right balance exists you do not experience tooth decay. Unfortunately, there are a great many ways to upset the natural balance of dental health and each leads to tooth decay and gum disease.

Sugar, that great dietary evil we keep hearing about, does play a role in tooth decay, just not the one that you believe. Your teeth do not rot in the presence of sugar; it is merely food for the bacteria in your mouth and causes major explosions in their population. There is scientific research demonstrating how sugar actually influences tooth decay and it is likely that you have never heard about this stunning information.

Would you be surprised to learn that there are people whose teeth are coated with plaque, rarely brush their teeth, and yet have no tooth decay? On the other hand, there are people who brush, floss, and rinse religiously and are plagued with dental problems. What would account for such a paradox, and is there an answer that can help you?

The real truth about tooth decay, gum disease, and the degenerative diseases that are caused by poor oral health, is more complex than you would think. Are you aware that your teeth have the ability to defend against the harsh, bacteria infested conditions in your mouth?

Barring external factors that may break or fracture your teeth, they are designed to remain healthy. There is a way to switch off the ability of your teeth to maintain their strong healthy state, and once this biological switch is flipped to the off position the process of destruction sets in. Odds are that most people reading this book have already unintentionally switched off the ability of their teeth to stay healthy.

Depending on how much damage has already been done to your teeth, you can take corrective measures that will be beneficial in nearly all situations. Children in particular will benefit when parents understand and enforce the knowledge gained from reading this material. The benefit for adults can be substantial as well, though in cases where there is already major trauma from decay and dental procedures, the struggle to maintain dental health will be more of a challenge.

As you read this book, keep the following three points in mind and think about how you can make choices that will have a positive beneficial outcome:

1. You can brush and floss your teeth several times every day and still get cavities and gum disease. Bushing and flossing are necessary, but not enough to protect your dental and physical health. Until the day you die, billions of bacteria in your mouth will always be actively looking to feed and breed; the decisions you make each day will determine the degree to which the bacteria are symbiotic or destructive. You will always be at risk for dental problems,

but making the right choices on a daily basis can dramatically reduce the risk. Even if you are in a state of chronically poor health, you can learn how to manage the bacteria and minimize their damage to your gums and teeth.

2. Tooth decay and gum disease can be prevented with the right cleaning regimen and dietary adjustments. Remember, bacteria will always exist in your mouth. The only "cure" would be to permanently destroy all the bacteria in your mouth, and we know that is not going to happen unless a specific vaccination is developed to make you immune to the exact bacteria that are responsible for gum disease. The objective in this book is to teach you how to make the right dietary adjustments to strengthen your natural ability to manage bacteria, and effectively keep bacterial populations in check with simple, inexpensive products that are commonly available.

3. There are consequences for failing to take responsibility for your dental health. Gum disease and tooth decay have been linked with heart disease, diabetes, dementia, and other chronic diseases. Yes, poor dental health can contribute to life-altering diseases. This book is about more than preventing tooth decay and gum loss. It is about maintaining your overall health and preventing your lack of oral health from contributing to even more serious health conditions.

I hope that you will take the time to implement the simple suggestions in this book. By all means, please consult your dentist or physician for additional guidance and information. There is no substitute for obtaining proper medical attention from a qualified health professional. Now, it is important for you to understand that tooth decay and gum disease have far more dangerous outcomes than losing teeth, and we will discuss this in the next chapter.

The Connection Between Tooth Decay and Degenerative Disease

Research studies have disclosed a link between periodontal disease and stroke, cancer, arthritis, dementia, pulmonary disease, and other diseases. The Journal of The American Dental Association in its August 2009 Volume 140, published information about the correlation between root canals and coronary heart disease. During their research study the ADA found a significant relationship between reported root canals and heart disease.

Unfortunately, many people have taken this information as an indication that having a root canal can lead to heart disease. When the pulp of your tooth becomes infected, bacteria are released directly into your bloodstream by the blood vessels within the tooth's pulp. Basically, the damage to your internal organs is well underway before the root canal takes place. The same bacteria found in an infected mouth can also be found in arterial plaque.

In May 2008, the American Association for Cancer Research issued a public release - http://www.eurekalert.org/pub_releases/2008-05/aafctls051308.php - about the results of a study conducted by Japanese researchers on several thousand patients. The researchers measured the rates of various cancers to the rates of tooth loss in cancer patients, and compared the results with thousands of study participants who did not have cancer. Their study indicated that people suffering tooth loss were 136 percent more likely to develop esophageal cancer, had a 68 percent higher possibility of having head and neck cancer, and a 58 percent higher chance of developing lung cancer. Basically, the study found a proportionally higher cancer risk associated with higher rates of tooth loss.

The Journal of the American Dental Association reported in its October 2007 vol. 138 issue that there is a potential risk of developing dementia associated with dental disease. In a decade long aging and Alzheimer disease study involving 144 Nuns, researchers found that participants with the fewest teeth also had the highest rate of dementia. Since the primary mechanism involved in tooth loss is tooth decay, it is easy to see the importance of prevention through diet and diligent oral care.

Celiac disease is commonly associated with gluten intolerance, however there is also a connection involving your teeth. The National Institutes of Health reports that that Celiac disease can affect development of teeth, enamel pitting, and discoloration. There is a good chance that dental problems associated with Celiac disease are symptomatic of high levels of phytic acid present in grains. Phytic acid is essentially an antinutrient and is predominately eaten in the form of bread and other whole grains; phytic acid is present in the bran of practically all grains.

In your digestive tract, phytic acid binds to important minerals such as calcium, magnesium, iron, and zinc, rendering those vitamins insoluble and indigestible in your intestinal tract. A diet high in grains reduces the bioavailable minerals needed for the development and maintenance of your bones and teeth. Most of the phytic acid in grains can be neutralized by soaking for several hours before processing, but soaking is not part of the commercial process of manufacturing grain-based products.

Decaying teeth can lead to fatal brain infection as bacteria flood into your bloodstream. It is not uncommon for people to die as a result of abscessed teeth. In order to learn how to prevent tooth decay and gum disease it is important that you learn why teeth decay, and that is the subject of the next chapter.

Why Your Teeth Decay

Far too many people expend a great deal of effort brushing, flossing, and rinsing, and still have to endure bleeding gums and tooth decay. The objective here is to help you gain an understanding of the real causes of dental problems so that you will have a logical basis for performing self-treatment rather than just taking advice on faith. Understanding the fundamental cause of tooth decay involves learning why a failing fluid transport system inside of your teeth, and acid in your mouth, are the primary factors behind gum disease and decaying teeth. We will discuss the importance of the circulatory system inside teeth and what causes fluid transport failure. In addition, you are going to learn that there are several independent elements that cause an acidic state in your mouth. You are probably strongly objecting to the exclusion of bacteria from the dental health equation, and yes they do play their role, but just not the one you may believe.

Certain conditions must exist in your mouth before bacteria become a dental problem. Bacterial activity leading to tooth decay and gum disease is part of the symptom, not the cause, of dental problems. Oral bacteria actually help prevent germs from entering your digestive tract and causing disease. Without bacteria in your oral cavity, you would soon suffer from an overgrowth of fungus and be open to far more germ infections. These germs enter your mouth from the air and the many things you put into your mouth every day. So, as shocking as it may seem, the bacteria in your mouth are actually good for you. It is in your mouth where your bacteria successfully do battle with these pathogenic invaders and become the first line of defense for your immune system.

It is very important for you to understand that stopping dental disease is not a simple issue of fixing one problem and you are done. We will address each of the most important issues to give you a comprehensive understanding of the root cause of tooth decay and gum disease. Once you know why problems occur, you will be better equipped to take your role as an active participant in improving and maintaining your dental health. Below is a summary of four major factors leading to dental disease; we will discuss each of these factors in greater detail in following chapters.

1. You may not realize that your teeth have their own circulatory system that moves nutrients into your teeth and removes waste. Each tooth is a living organ that is designed to successfully exist within the hostile environment of your mouth. You have the ability to halt the normal biological functions in your teeth, and you will learn what you have probably already done to cause this problem. When the natural metabolic process of your teeth is interrupted, your teeth lose their natural ability to maintain their health and that is when tooth decay can begin. According to scientific research, the flow of fluids within the tooth structure can be

altered, thus setting up your teeth for certain decay. In the next chapter titled, "The Fluid Transport System Inside Your Teeth", we will discuss the very important cause and effect factors in play that determine the health of your teeth.

2. It is very important that you understand the role of PH (power of hydrogen) in relation to your dental and physical health and why you should avoid playing PH Roulette by following popular advice about manipulating the alkaline state of your body. There are measures you should take to help maintain a normal PH balance that do not include radical, unproven experiments that could damage your health. Information about the role of PH is discussed in the "Playing PH Roulette" chapter.

3. Next, we will take a brief look at the difference in dental disease between developed societies and less developed cultures. It is not at all unusual for less technologically developed societies to often have little, or no dental disease, even when they do not brush their teeth. Diet plays a definite part in this discrepancy, but simply extrapolating a simple solution based on dietary differences is another common mistake made by people looking for easy solutions to dental disease. The chapter covering this information is titled "Sources Of Acid Erosion" and you will begin to understand another factor in explaining why dental disease plagues modern civilizations. You will learn why and how your mouth becomes an acid-producing factory. Understanding how acidity triggers the production of undesirable bacterial conditions will help you be more determined to put a stop to this problem.

4. Finally, you will learn about the function of diet and the impact it has on the dental demineralization and remineralization process constantly taking place within your mouth. You will also learn that instead of resorting to radical dietary adventures, all you have to do is follow a few common sense eating rules.

The Fluid Transport System Inside Your Teeth

It is too easy to forget that the teeth in your mouth are far more than a collection of little rocks. Each tooth is a living organ and your body does its best to nurture teeth internally, and renew your tooth enamel with the minerals delivered by your salivary system. Few people know that there is a circulatory system within each tooth that, when functioning properly, does an amazing job of keeping the tooth healthy and preventing bacteria from invading.

In healthy teeth, fluids flow from inside the pulp of your teeth through the dentin, and out of the enamel into your mouth. Sounds crazy, right? Well there is scientific proof that this is a fact, and understanding that the flow of fluids in your teeth can be reversed is a major step in understanding why tooth decay is so difficult to prevent.

When the fluid pressure in your teeth is focused from inside to outside, bacteria have a much more difficult time penetrating the tooth. Once the fluid pressure in a tooth is reversed, lactic acid can easily accumulate on and inside your teeth, contributing to demineralization, and this opens the way for bacterial infection starting with tooth decay. Knowing what triggers the reversal of fluid pressure is one of the major keys to maintaining both your dental and physical health.

Dr. Ralph R Steinman and Dr. John Leonora proved through research on rats and pigs that fluid within teeth moves with an outward pressure through tooth dentin and enamel. You may want to read some of this research for yourself. A good summary was written by Dr. Ken Southward titled *The Systemic Theory of Dental Caries*, featured in General Dentistry, September/October 2011 Pg. 367-373 (www.agd.org/publications/articles/?ArtID=9892), and research by Steinman and Leonora, *Relationship of Fluid Transport Through the Dentin to the Incidence of Dental Caries*, is available in PDF file format at http://dr-jacques-imbeau.com/PDF/Dentinal%20fluid%20transport%20and%20caries.pdf.

Steinman and Leonora proved, in a study on rats, that the movement of fluid within the tooth could be stopped by the consumption of a high sucrose diet. Once the tooth's ability to circulate nutrients and remove waste has been compromised, plaque can easily accumulate and the tooth is more susceptible to acid demineralization.

Steinman and Leonora found that sugar impacts the hypothalamus, a small portion of the brain that controls many critical bodily functions. In a healthy state, the hypothalamus secretes a hormone that stimulates a large salivary gland known as the parotid gland. When stimulated by the hypothalamus, the parotid gland secretes a hormone that activates fluid movement within your teeth. Sugar is the primary culprit that short circuits the hormonal signals to your teeth, effectively inhibiting their natural ability to defend themselves by performing their normal metabolic activity.

There are people whose teeth are covered with plaque, rarely brush, and amazingly have no tooth decay. Although the dental community rarely acknowledges that dental plaque can exist without accompanying tooth decay, mention of this paradox is found in published accounts. One example of scholarly material identifying dental plaque occurring without the presence of tooth decay is from *A Survey of the Literature of Dental Caries, Publication 225 National Academy of Sciences - National Research Council 1952, Page 10, "Among more primitive people without the regular modern daily cleaning of the teeth, including those who have an extremely low incidence of caries, it is common to find heavy, tenacious plaque covering most of the crown. Nevertheless, after scraping off the debris, the enamel may have the most lustrous appearance."*

On the other hand, there are a great many people who brush, floss, use disinfecting rinses, and are still plagued with dental problems. It is highly probable that the explanation for this seeming paradox is twofold: the role that sugar plays in suppressing the secretion of hormones that activate the desirable metabolic process in your teeth, and the manner in which you eat sugar.

According to research, how dietary sugar is consumed is an important link in reducing the probability of tooth decay. In the *Proceedings of the Nutrition Society (1984), 43, 257-263, Nutrition and Dental Decay, By M. N. Naylord, Department of Periodontology and Preventive Dentistry*, human studies indicate that it is partially a timing issue; it is a matter of when you choose to eat sugar that has a direct influence on the development of tooth decay. People in the study who consumed sugar only with meals experienced dramatically fewer problems with tooth decay than people who eat sugary foods between meals.

At this point, a likely explanation for the plaque paradox exists for two reasons. First, it is possible to have plaque structures on tooth enamel that do not demineralize teeth when there is little, or no sugar present in your diet. Without sugar, it is difficult for bacteria to metabolize enough lactic acid to dissolve your tooth enamel. More important, a persistent lack of dietary sugar allows the fluid pressure in teeth to be maintained, effectively promoting internal tooth health while resisting acid and bacterial intrusion into the enamel surface.

The actual process of tooth decay begins before the appearance of your first cavity. Once a tooth's normal metabolic processes are switched off, acid produced by bacteria, acidic food, and acidic beverages begin demineralization of tooth enamel. After pores are open within the enamel, bacteria set up colonies protected from brushing, flossing, and rinsing, and the decay cycles gets underway in earnest. When the fluid pressure in teeth is activated, teeth are more resistant to invasion as long as there are no enamel fractures, and your teeth are not broken or chipped. In essence, the health of individual teeth is directly related to a lack of dietary sugar and the absence of acidic conditions associated with the consumption of sugar.

Understanding the variables involved in dental disease helps make sense of why the severity of tooth decay can be so dramatically different in human populations. When and how you consume sugar, whether you engage in a consistent dental hygiene regimen, and whether you engage in physical activities that can fracture or break teeth (cracking ice with your teeth), all play a role in the state of your dental health.

Considering the dramatic effect of sugar on the metabolic process in teeth, what other consequences are there that you may be suffering? Everyone seems to know that you should not consume too much sugar, now you have a specific reason as to why sugar has an impact on your health. After your teeth are compromised, bacteria invade the tooth pulp and are carried away to other organs in your body, setting the stage for a variety of degenerative diseases. Even the infamous abscessed tooth can cause brain damage, coma, and heart damage. Tragically, every year people die from infections directly related to abscessed teeth. Is sugar really worth the risk?

Sad to say, but most people will ignore this information on the premise that they consume little sugar. If you are eating the typical industrialized diet you are consuming huge amounts of sugar hidden in nearly every processed food you eat. Unless you prepare your own food from whole meat and vegetables, and ignore the canned and prepared foods in the center grocery aisles, you are consuming an amazing amount of sugar. Add to that the deliberate consumption of sugary treats and you have performed a major chemical change in your body.

Naturally, the question will arise, how much sugar is too much? You may as well ask, how much arsenic should you consume in small doses, or what is the safe dosage for human consumption of rat poison? Do yourself and your children a favor by doing some honest research and see how many health benefits are conferred by eating sugar. Will you be one of the many that choose to ignore scientific evidence about the impact of sugar on human health?

Take a little time to check the food labels on the products in your kitchen cabinets. Practically all of your food will have sugar or products labeled with an ingredient that ends with "ose", as in fructose sugar. It is very likely that close to 100% of the sugars hidden in your food are derived from genetically altered plants. Do a little research about genetically modified food and you may strengthen your motivation to avoid running an unproven, untested chemical experiment on your body.

In addition to risking your dental health, excessive sugar consumption will help tilt your body toward acidosis, the condition associated with the PH of your blood being too low. Sadly, many people are under the impression that they can self-medicate to control the PH of their saliva and blood.

Playing PH Roulette

It is pretty easy to encounter helpful advice regarding the PH of your saliva and your body. The current theory is that your body can become so acidic that your saliva will begin to demineralize your teeth and, to counter that problem, you just need to follow the right health program and balance the PH in your body. One of the main problems with this theory is that saliva PH and blood PH do not correlate very well; there are many factors that will cause wide swings in saliva PH while blood PH remains relatively unchanged.

You can easily find a wealth of dietary products, books, courses, and advisers selling you a magic pill or method to help you adjust your blood PH and neutralize your saliva PH. Normalizing blood PH happens to be something that your body already does quite well on its own without the interference of health gurus. According to widely available information, you simply perform a litmus test of your saliva or urine to determine if you are in a neutral or slightly alkaline state. If you are in an acidic state, typical advice is to begin taking a variety of supplements and/or make radical dietary changes. There are many problems with this simplistic approach, the least of which is that such advice is likely to have very little effect on your oral PH, and you are running a potentially dangerous chemical experiment on your body without actually knowing what your blood PH really is.

The only accurate way to measure blood PH is with a blood test. Saliva and urine tests only tell you what the PH is for your saliva or urine and there are a great many factors that cause those PH tests to vary widely from a blood PH test. Many factors influence the PH of the saliva in your mouth including the consumption of pharmaceutical drugs, how clean your mouth is, or whether you have an existing pathological health condition. Saliva tends to remain in a narrow PH range, typically on the slightly acidic side, and usually does not fall below 6.3 PH due to the presence of phosphate and bicarbonate in your saliva, which help neutralize acid.

There are a few things you need to understand about the PH of your body and how it relates to your dental health and overall physical condition. Your body has systems that keep your blood in a narrow PH range of 7.35 to 7.45. Regardless of what you eat, you have three major systems actively working to keep your blood in an alkaline state. These important systems go to extraordinary lengths to maintain an alkaline PH and consist of the Buffer System (Carbonic Acid-Bicarbonate Buffer System, Protein Buffer System, and Phosphate Buffer System), your kidneys working to eliminate hydrogen ions, and your lungs working to eliminate carbon dioxide.

Even if you are a smoker, drink alcohol regularly, and have abused your body with highly processed foods, it is likely that your blood PH is in its normal range. With enough abuse these critical PH buffering systems can and will fail. Although blood PH is a very important factor that can influence your dental health, it falls way short on the scale of issues that directly impact your dental health. Once your blood PH falls much below a PH of 7.35, dental issues will be the least of your health problems.

Keeping your lungs, kidneys, and buffer system healthy is the best way to avoid disrupting your normal blood PH balance. Three of the easiest ways to protect these vital systems are to avoid smoking, limit alcohol consumption to very moderate amounts, and eat a healthy balanced diet consisting primarily of unprocessed foods. The term "unprocessed foods" has to do with foods that have not been altered by a manufacturing process where you are eating out of a box, can, or precooked meals. Nearly all of the food items located in the center aisles of grocery stores are processed and will have a negative impact on your physical and mental health.

It is not necessary to consume exotic supplements, or run a chemical experiment with fasting, detox, or an extreme vegan diet to maintain a healthy blood PH. Of greater concern is the PH condition in your mouth, how long it stays in an acidic state, and what you can do to keep your oral PH more neutral. The role that oral acidic conditions play in undermining your dental health is the topic of the next chapter.

Sources of Acid Erosion

Acid and Your Teeth

The enamel coating on your teeth is one of the hardest substances in your body and is mostly composed of crystalline calcium phosphate formed into a structure of enamel rods. What is really amazing is that your enamel surface is constantly being replaced to a limited degree by the minerals in your saliva. Unfortunately, in the presence of excessive wear, or acidic conditions, your tooth enamel can be damaged to such an extent that it no longer protects the vulnerable layers of dentine and pulp.

You may not realize that there are micropores in tooth enamel leading to the inner part of your teeth. Once the pores are opened, your teeth become sensitive to cold and heat and this is often the first sign for many people that their tooth enamel has been damaged. During an extended acidic cycle, the PH in your mouth does not have a chance to return to neutral and your saliva will not be able to remineralize the exposed micropores. Bacteria begin to populate the open pores and form plaque if they are not removed through brushing or disinfection. Once plaque is formed, the bacteria soon go into an anaerobic state and excrete lactic acid as part of their metabolic process, effectively beginning the cycle of tooth decay.

The primary sources of acid that damage tooth enamel include:

- Acidic food and beverages
- Acid reflux
- Frequent vomiting - bulimia
- Mature dental plaque biofilm
- Acidic teeth whitening products

It is very common for a person to have multiple sources of acid present in their mouth during the course of one day. With each acid exposure, tooth enamel is softened for a period of time. The longer and more frequent the acid exposure, the faster tooth enamel will soften and dissolve. With repeated acid exposure your teeth can be damaged to an irreversible level, and this does not include acid produced by bacterial colonization.

Soon after your teeth are bathed in acid, your saliva works to wash away and neutralize acid back to a level where tooth enamel remineralization begins. Minerals are delivered to your teeth through saliva as part of your body's natural defense against acid and bacteria; this keeps minerals in tooth enamel from being leeched until your teeth are destroyed. Saliva delivers the materials needed to keep your tooth enamel repaired and the best way to insure that it does its job is to maintain the rest of your body in a good state of health. After you stop eating and drinking acidic foods or beverages, your saliva's PH neutralizing and remineralization process will take at least thirty minutes to an hour to normalize; until then it is not safe to brush your teeth. Your tooth enamel becomes soft early in the acidification phase and is vulnerable to damage from brushing, so it is always a good idea to wait awhile before you brush your teeth.

Acidic Foods and Beverages

One of the most likely explanations for the difference between the dental disease epidemic of modern civilization, compared to isolated people who are relatively free of dental disease, lies in understanding how and what we eat. As an example, Dr. Weston Price located a group of isolated people in Switzerland whose diet was primarily based on raw dairy products, whole rye bread, and limited quantities of potatoes, green foods, and some meat from sheep. This isolated group of people had an extremely low rate of dental problems. Essentially, these Swiss people consumed a diet that possess acid buffering characteristics which is high in calcium, fat-soluble vitamins, and minerals.

In contrast, more advanced civilizations consume a diet rich in carbohydrates, acidic foods, and corrosive beverages. The key factor is that modernized people eat in such a way that their teeth are constantly bathed with acid producing food and drink, with a significant portion of the consumption being in the form of complex carbohydrates. It just so happens that oral bacteria love to feed on carbohydrates and the result is a massive population boom of lactic acid producing bacteria. The modern mouth rarely has time to balance PH levels before more acid is ingested.

Modern people tend to engage in eating patterns that maintain a constant acidic condition in the mouth. Keeping the mouth in a highly acidic state for prolonged time periods continually softens and erodes tooth enamel. In short order, even with consistent brushing and flossing, bacteria invade enamel micropores and decay sets in. To make matters worse, most people in the civilized world worry little about regularly cleaning their teeth until pain begins.

Destroying Your Teeth One Sip and One Bite At A Time

As a baseline to understand the significance of PH in your mouth, normal saliva will have a PH somewhere around 6.3 to 7.0 and **Battery Acid has a PH of 1.0**. Keeping in mind that **minerals in your tooth enamel begin to dissolve at a PH of 5.0 to 5.5 and lower**, here is how you destroy your teeth:

Constantly sipping the following, or similar beverages throughout the day (Note that no product names are mentioned as I do not want the long arm and deep pockets of legal departments at corporate manufacturers after me).

- Bottled and canned soft drinks PH - 2.4 to 3.0
- Diet sodas PH - 2.4 to 3.0
- Boxed and Bottled Fruit Juices - 2.4 to 4.3
- Sports Drinks - 2.4 to 3.4

- Energy Drinks   - 2.6 to 3.9
- Lime and Lemon Juice - 2.0 to 2.6
- Canned Cranberry Juice - 2.3 to 2.5
- Canned Grapefruit Juice - 2.9 to 3.3
- Canned Pineapple Juice - 3.3 to 3.6
- Processed Orange Juice - 3.3 to 4.2

Whether at home, work, or play, a substantial population of adults and children spend their day guzzling an array of beverages promoted by advertisers as being energizing, healthy, and rehydrating. Many of these beverages are in fact toxic in addition to being highly acidic. When you spend your day constantly refreshing yourself with the types of drinks listed above, you are slowly poisoning your body and destroying your teeth.

The modern civilization attack on teeth consists of all day consumption of candy, cookies, donuts, chewing gum (with sugar), cake, chips, and other highly refined acidic carbohydrates. Most of these snacks are eaten with, before, and after acidic beverages. As you chew, the junk foods are broken down into a paste and this paste coats your teeth, mouth, and tongue, leaving huge amounts of food for bacteria to eat. A literal explosion of bacterial populations will occur, along with their metabolic waste product known as lactic acid. So, we ingest beverages that are not too far off the acid scale from battery acid, consume food that is acidic, all of which keep the PH in the mouth at the wrong level, and then bacteria do their part by consuming the sugar and other carbohydrates in your mouth to produce plenty of additional acid. The cycle continues all day long and the saliva in your mouth has no chance of overcoming this acid tsunami.

Many people compound the problem by aggressively brushing their softened teeth and unintentionally cause even more damage to their teeth. To make matters worse after brushing, they immediately begin consuming acidic drinks and junk food, thinking that they have properly cared for their teeth. This constant acidic state in the mouth sets the stage for destructive demineralization of tooth enamel, and offers very little chance for teeth to be remineralized.

At this point, a picture should be beginning to emerge as to why there are major differences between the isolated Swiss people and their modern counterparts. Also keep in mind that within modern societies there is a significant population of people who have little to no dental disease.

People in our more advanced civilizations who have few dental problems will tend to eat and drink differently than their diseased neighbors. They will mostly be eating whole foods in lieu of highly processed meals, drink beverages that are far less corrosive than soft drinks, do not snack on highly processed carbohydrates all day, and as a result of their habits, permit a more neutral PH state to exist in their mouth so that normal tooth enamel remineralization can occur. When these people regularly engage in brushing and flossing, their dental health is far better than the average person in modern civilization.

Another factor that allows the modern person to

experience good dental health is not using their teeth as a tool for anything other than eating normal food. The primary factor in dental failure for our ancestors was their tendency to use their teeth as tools to crack nuts, bones, grind hard grains, soften hard fibrous plant foods, chew animal hides, and crush grit and dirt in their food. Of course, many of us make the same mistakes by crushing ice, hard candy, and chewing objects such as toothpicks or pencils. Tooth enamel is hard, but brittle; once it is fractured, or broken, a perfect place is formed for bacteria to colonize and set up the anaerobic lactic acid production cycle resulting in tooth decay.

Our ancestors cleaned their teeth with sticks and straw, if at all. Most primitive people were able to maintain strong healthy teeth if they did not suffer tooth enamel destruction from grinding, fracture, or breaking. The food they ate was usually whole food that, when chewed, still remained in relatively large particles that were nearly all swallowed. The remainder of large pieces of food either dislodged on their own, or the person removed them by picking at their teeth. For the most part, primitive people were able to maintain a low acid state in their mouth where the dominant process was tooth enamel remineralization. The predominate process in the mouth of modern man is dental demineralization.

Ancient societies that cultivated grains tended to experience much higher levels of tooth decay. Most likely, their higher incidence of tooth decay had to do with the consumption of complex carbohydrates and the antinutrient properties of phytic acid in grain.

Acid Reflux and Your Teeth

Acid reflux is when stomach contents pass through your lower esophageal sphincter into your esophagus. With a PH of 2.0 the reflux of stomach materials is highly corrosive. If you suffer from acid reflux, your teeth are at highest risk of damage at night when stomach contents may escape all the way through your esophagus into your mouth. Compounding the problem is the fact that at night saliva flow in your mouth nearly halts and this creates an environment ripe for significant mineral leeching from tooth enamel.

Acid reflux disease, also known as gastroesophageal reflux disease (GERD), can be caused by a hiatal hernia. More commonly, acid reflux will be triggered by obesity, overeating, or eating certain foods such as garlic, tomatoes, food cooked in highly processed vegetable oil, spicy foods, drinking alcohol or carbonated beverages, and other dietary contaminants.

I suffered with severe acid reflux for several years and consumed up to two large bottles of antacids each week. The permanent solution to getting rid of indigestion and acid reflux for me was when I eliminated highly processed complex carbohydrates and commercial cooking oils. The very worst items in my diet were processed flour products (white or whole grain), cooked or served with foods containing vegetable oils or margarine.

Unless you have a hiatal hernia, acid reflux should be nearly 100% preventable with dietary modifications. There will be information about recommended dietary adjustments in a later chapter.

The problem with chronic acid reflux is that not only do you risk extensive damage to your teeth, you are also subject to mild acidosis with a subsequent acid build up in your pancreas and kidneys, putting you at risk of diabetes and kidney stones. In addition, the excess acid can cause bone calcium to be lost making you more susceptible to osteoporosis.

Vomiting And Your Teeth

People who frequently vomit due to the side effects of chemotherapy, various disease states, or bulimia, are subject to massive damage to their tooth structure. One of the worst things you can do is brush your teeth immediately after you have thrown up; the bristles of your toothbrush can literally use the acid to scrub away tooth enamel.

To protect your teeth after vomiting, immediately rinse your mouth with fresh water then dissolve 1/2 teaspoon baking soda in half a cup of water. Use the baking soda mixture as an acid neutralizing mouthwash. Wait at least an hour before brushing your teeth.

Mature Dental Plaque Biofilm

So exactly what is a dental plaque biofilm? It is simply a way of describing a colony of bacteria. There are hundreds of different strains of bacteria in your mouth at any one time. Depending on how clean you keep your mouth, the overall population of bacteria in your mouth alone can exceed the entire human population on earth.

If your mouth is very clean, a sizable portion of the bacteria in your mouth will be free-floating and waiting to attach to a surface. Once attached to your tooth enamel, compatible bacteria form into a mushroom shaped microcolony that has its own ecosystem. Each bacterial microcolony may have its own unique combination of bacterial species.

Within a few seconds of cleaning your teeth thoroughly, glycoproteins in your saliva begin attaching to tooth enamel and form a protein film called a pellicle formation. The purpose of this protein film is to initially protect the enamel and help with remineralization. Bacteria floating through your saliva attach to the pellicle formation, other nearby bacteria, and begin to grow hair like structures that attract more bacteria. As the bacteria attach, they excrete a protective slime layer effectively anchoring the growth to the tooth surface. Once the tooth surface is coated with bacteria, they begin multiplying outward into mushroom shaped micro colonies. Rapid growth begins as additional bacteria attach to each other and begin linking colonies into a plaque formation.

As the plaque biofilm begins to mature, lactic acid is excreted in concentrated areas when bacteria feed on carbohydrates siphoned to them through fluid channels within the colony; the lactic acid then begins to demineralize tooth enamel. The dissolved areas are rooted by additional bacterial growth, which leads to more lactic acid dissolving your teeth in a cycle called tooth decay.

Plaque formations begin to wedge open the area between gum tissue and the base of your teeth, leading to swelling and further bacterial intrusion into the region below your gum line. Once a subgingival (below the gum line) area has been populated by bacterial colonies, they are relatively protected and resistant to cleaning and antibiotics. Mature plaque colonies generally can only be removed by more aggressive dental procedures performed by your dentist.

In the early stages of gum disease, a dentist can remove the plaque formations below your gum line by a process called scaling. Your dentist will use a hand scaler or ultrasonic tip to scrape the bacterial colonies from the tooth surface. Later stages of periodontal disease require a surgical procedure to remove the plaque.

By far, the easiest solution is to never allow plaque biofilm to develop beyond the initial attachment, or immature colonization phase. Unfortunately, brushing and flossing are no guarantee that you will be successful since neither can disturb bacteria growing in deeper gingival crevices at the edge of your teeth and gums.

Acidic Teeth Whitening Products

Hollywood has motivated tens of thousands of people to go for that gleaming white smile. Unfortunately, it is all too easy to unintentionally abuse teeth whitening products and cause irreversible gum damage, permanent loss of tooth enamel, or both. Either outcome can lead to significant dental problems you would rather avoid.

Even teeth whitening procedures carried out by a dentist may carry a significant risk. Dissolving tooth enamel to remove stains is a common procedure that exposes the micropores in your teeth to bacterial colonization. Human teeth naturally have a slight yellowish tinge. Tooth enamel is somewhat translucent and this allows the color of the yellowish colored dentin beneath to shade tooth color. Brilliant white teeth are unnatural for adults.

Diet and Dental Health

Medical professionals have sought answers to the mystery of tooth decay by visiting people living in remote, non-industrialized areas. Often these isolated people have very little tooth decay or gum disease, and enjoy a robust state of health compared to modernized societies. It is wise to learn the valuable dietary lessons from the studies made with these people. The temptation is to make simplistic dietary extrapolations, based on a study of what a tribe's primitive diet may have been, and this can be a mistake. While it is true that many less developed people eating a diet high in animal protein and fat have few dental problems, and some primitive vegetarian cultures also experienced low rates of dental decay, is it really necessary to attempt to replicate such a diet?

If bacteria are found in the mouths of all humans, and some groups of people have little to no tooth decay while other people have substantial decay, then it should make sense that some factor other than bacteria is most likely the primary cause of dental disease. Some groups of our ancestors used their teeth in ways that guaranteed erosion from chewing hard dietary fiber, grit, and using their teeth as a tool. Once their teeth were fractured and broken, bacterial invasion into damaged enamel began along with subsequent tooth decay. Other primitive ancestors did not use their teeth as tools and suffered far fewer dental problems. Likewise, substantial numbers of modern people who do not physically abuse their teeth get to enjoy very little tooth decay while eating a wide variety of foods made available by improved agricultural practices.

There are many factors that influence dental health including stress, malnourishment, famine, disease, and trauma to teeth from dietary and external abuse. Many of these factors are beyond our ability to control. We are able to learn valuable lessons by comparing what we eat, and how we eat, to less modernized people who have few dental problems. One such lesson may be learned by the observations Dr. Weston Price made while visiting people living in an isolated valley in Switzerland. Dr. Price noted that the inhabitants had an extremely low incidence of tooth decay while subsisting primarily on a diet of raw milk, and raw milk products such as cheese, cream, and butter. There is scientific evidence of a strong correlation between tooth enamel remineralization, bacterial suppression, and the consumption of hard and soft cheese. The diet consumed by the Swiss people observed by Dr. Price was also very high in fat-soluble vitamins and minerals.

Diet is one of those subjects that attract controversy and discord. Depending on whom you talk to, what book you read, or health professional you consult, it is extremely likely that you will receive diverse, polarized opinions that enter the realm of dogma. Most everyone reading this chapter will likely be firmly entrenched in their idea of proper diet, so the information presented about diet will be confined to just a few major points that are important. Just keep an open mind and perhaps this chapter may help you.

There are dietary plans out there that claim amazing results in reversing gum disease and remineralization of dental cavities if you follow the diet. Although there are claims that cavities can heal on their own with the right diet, I have not found any verifiable evidence that a cavity can repair itself through dietary adjustments once tooth enamel has been penetrated and a cavity has formed. No doubt, what you eat will play an important role in your dental and overall physical health, and I am a strong advocate for eating the freshest organic foods available. However, relying solely on diet to remedy your dental problems is likely to be a very big mistake.

If you do not follow a regular plan to clean and sanitize your teeth, gums, and mouth, you are still at risk of developing some form of dental disease regardless of the purity of your diet. The simple fact is that no program or diet can guarantee that you will not ever experience gum disease or tooth decay. However, when you match a good diet with the right dental cleaning regimen, you will be able to lower your risk of incurring dental problems to the absolute minimum.

You should consider the dietary element of your life to be the base that supports your immune system and revitalizes your cells with vitamins, minerals, and enzymes that support your life energy. The natural healing processes of your body need to be supplemented by your active participation in a systematic daily program to clean your teeth.

The Importance of Diet and Saliva

One of the most important elements necessary for your dental health is the health of your saliva. According to the American Dental Association, "Saliva is like a bloodstream to the mouth." Phosphate and calcium ions are deposited by saliva onto the surface of your teeth. Over a long period of time, where tooth enamel remineralization exceeds demineralization, the enamel will get harder and more durable. For this important mineralization process to happen at optimal levels, your body needs to be able to release sufficient quantities of necessary minerals into your saliva and your diet plays an important role in this function.

Unfortunately, due to the consumption of highly processed foods, significant groups of people are experiencing demineralization leading to bone loss and tooth decay. One of the major dietary factors that determine whether your body can regulate the calcium and phosphorus levels necessary for bone mineralization is the presence of calcitriol, a steroid hormone.

Calcitriol - Vitamin D3 and Diet

Calcitriol, also known as Vitamin D3, is a steroid hormone important in your bone mineralization process. People who receive adequate amounts of D3 generally experience much better dental health than people who are chronically deficient. This important vitamin facilitates the absorption and delivery of phosphate and calcium into your saliva.

A wide variety of cells in your body contain receptors for vitamin D3. The importance of D3 cannot be underestimated since it is critical in modulating cell growth, reducing inflammation, promoting neuromuscular and immune functions, and other critical processes regulating cell proliferation, differentiation, and cell elimination.

There are a limited number of sources where you can obtain Vitamin D3. Unfortunately many people take a poor substitute in the form of vitamin D2 supplements. The very best source of Vitamin D3 is that which your body processes when your skin gets adequate exposure to sunlight. If you receive sufficient sunlight you will not need additional supplementation.

Most people in modern civilization do not get the amount of sunlight needed to provide the quantity of D3 necessary for good health, and are forced to resort to supplementation. The amount of daily sunlight you need will vary depending upon the pigmentation in your skin. The more fair skinned you are, the less sunlight you require, with some people only needing 15 minutes or less.

The best dietary sources of Vitamin D3 include fatty fish such as salmon, tuna, and mackerel. Fish liver oils are another good dietary source for D3. Smaller amounts are available in egg yolks, beef liver, whole milk, and cheese. To get the very best dietary Vitamin D3 you should try to consume wild caught fish, eggs from free-range cage free chickens, grass fed beef that has not been treated with antibiotics and growth hormones, and cheese made from raw milk. Unfortunately, many of the people who need these whole foods the most can least afford the high cost. Even worse, they mostly consume a diet of highly processed carbohydrates and junk beverages. Even if you cannot afford organic eggs, dairy, produce, and meat, at least prepare your meals from whole food and avoid nearly all precooked foods that are ready to eat cold or warm.

Diet, Physical Health, and Dental Health

For your body to function at optimal levels you require high quality sources of minerals, protein, vitamins, and fat. In terms of vitamins, there are two important groups: fat soluble and water-soluble vitamins. Vegetarians will violently disagree with some of the views presented here concerning vitamins, and that is just fine. Every person must follow the conviction of his or her beliefs and do what they feel is in their best interest.

The very best sources of fat-soluble vitamins A, D, E, and K are from animals in the form of eggs, liver, fish oils, whole milk, and whole milk products such as butter and cheese. Generally, your body has to do less conversion to utilize the fat-soluble vitamins from animal sources. Sunlight synthesized by your skin is the very best source for vitamin D. These important vitamins are stored in your liver and released as needed. If you are eating a good diet, and get adequate sunshine, taking off-the-shelf vitamins to supplement vitamins A, D, E, and K is not a good idea and may lead to toxic side effects.

Vitamins C and B-Complex are water soluble, meaning that they are not stored in your body for later use and must be replaced as part of your daily diet. B-Complex vitamins are easily available from animal sources such as meat, fish, liver, whole milk, poultry, eggs, oysters, and shellfish. Some of the best commonly available sources of Vitamin C are red and green peppers, citrus fruits, dark leafy greens, broccoli, strawberries, melons, and tomatoes. Simply including a good variety of these vitamin sources in your daily diet will help keep you healthy.

Unless your physician has prescribed vitamin supplements, you will be better off not taking the supplements available at your local pharmacy, grocery, or discount stores. Many of these "vitamins" are synthetic isolates combined with other chemicals to mimic the action of real vitamins. In addition, artificial coloring in the form of dye is added to many of the most popular vitamin supplements on the market.

The dyes added to vitamin supplements, and significant numbers of food and beverage products, are known to be toxic. Most of these artificial colors are one form or another of Lake dye, a non-water soluble form of dye made by mixing with Aluminum Hydroxide. Lake dyes have been linked to behavioral problems in children and there is a risk of aluminum toxicity when consuming aluminum hydroxide from vitamins, food, and antacids. It is known that aluminum accumulates in tissues and organs resulting in their dysfunction and toxicity. Do some research on your own and you will likely agree that it is dangerous to consume many of the commercially prepared vitamin supplements.

Customizing Your Diet

Governments, most books, and health gurus generally promote a one-size-fits-all eating plan, while many researchers claim that individual nutritional requirements may be a function of genetic inheritance where people of different blood types have different dietary needs. One thing is for certain, we are all unique and have varying degrees of reaction to different foods. It is no secret that people from different parts of our world do not tolerate foods consumed by their counterparts on other parts of the planet.

From a nutritional standpoint, people are far more alike than they are different, however those small differences sometimes have devastating health consequences. You may want to conduct research into metabolic typing to see if you may benefit from the addition or elimination of certain foods. There is a free online test provided by Dr. Joseph Mercola located at http://products.mercola.com/nutritional-typing that may be a good starting point in your research.

Another major area of dietary disagreement is whether organic foods are any better than factory farm food. A review published in the American Journal of Clinical Nutrition claimed that organic food offers no better nutritionally related health benefits than conventional food. Unfortunately, as far as I can tell, that conclusion was not based on extensive scientific research and qualifies as more opinion than fact. The United States is currently engaged in a massive, untested chemical experiment on its population with its support of genetically modified food. Countries around the world are banning GMO foods. Although there are numerous clear warnings from scientists that planting genetically modified crops is a failing technology, US federal regulators push ahead to make GMO foods the law of the land. Nearly every processed packaged food in your local grocery includes some form of genetically modified food. My personal opinion is that consuming these polluted foods is a very dangerous way to experiment with your health.

Whether you eat organic or conventional factory food is certainly a matter of personal choice. I would personally encourage you to make it your goal to buy as much of your food as possible that is free of contaminants such as pesticides, herbicides, fungicides, antibiotics, hormones, toxic metals, and exotic chemical additives.

The most toxic food on the planet, and likely the root of the degenerative disease epidemic in the industrialized world, is found in the center aisles of grocery stores in the form of highly processed canned, boxed, and frozen meals. Even the whole foods that you cook and prepare at home are often polluted with toxic pesticides, herbicides, drugs, and hormones. Your best bet for quality food is local farmers.

Most communities have a farmers market where you can obtain fruit, vegetables, meat, eggs, and whole milk that has been produced by either safe organic methods, or growing practices that lead to more nutritious foods.

Government regulators will tell you that the amount of pesticides, herbicides, fungicides, and toxic metals present in processed foods is delivered in quantities deemed safe for human consumption. The lunacy behind this viewpoint is the belief that a little of something toxic will not harm you. The problem is that we do not just consume a small amount of one toxin every now and then. The reality is that we consume a large number of toxins several times a day for years from industrially processed foods and then are surprised that cancer and other degenerative diseases are reaching epidemic levels in the United States. It is true that eating a really teeny-tiny portion of rat poison may have no apparent effect on you. On the other side of the issue is the question of whether you would deliberately choose to eat weed killer in extremely small amounts? Would you deliberately eat small quantities of insect killer every day for years? Well, these poisons are included in nearly every processed food you consume.

Two good websites for food and health related information are http://www.naturalnews.com and http://www.mercola.com. I have no relationship with either of these websites, do not always agree with their point of view, and sometimes think their views are a little over the top. On the other hand, both websites do offer a wealth of solid health and diet insights that can be startling.

In addition to diet, it is important to refrain from activities that place your teeth in jeopardy. Let's take a look at all the easy ways you can damage your teeth.

Thirteen Ways To Destroy Your Teeth

Destroying your teeth is incredibly easy. Below is a list of common activities that can damage your teeth, your health, or both.

1. Brushing your teeth immediately after eating highly acidic food, drinking acidic beverages, or vomiting, is a poor idea. Extreme acid conditions in your mouth soften your tooth enamel and immediate brushing will help scrub the mineral layer from your teeth.

2. Your teeth were not designed for crushing hard objects. Whatever you put into your mouth should be soft enough that excessive force is not necessary to break the object into smaller pieces. Cracking ice, nuts, hard candy, and chewing on pencils, toothpicks, and other hard items can fracture or chip your teeth. The outer enamel on your teeth is not only very hard, it is also brittle and will break under pressure. If an item is too hard to crush easily, remove it from your mouth and do not risk permanent injury to your teeth.

3. Did you know that hot and cold temperatures could crack your teeth? Switching from eating something that is

extremely hot or cold to the opposite extreme temperature will fracture your teeth. It is likely that you may not even realize that the fracture has happened.

4. Never use your teeth to open objects. Your teeth are not suitable tools for pulling open stuck shoelaces, opening bottles, or biting through cans.

5. Mouth piercing usually involves the insertion of hard jewelry that can potentially break your teeth. Mouth jewelry also provides another nesting place for bacterial colonies to grow, safe from brushing.

6. Far too many people play contact sports without wearing a mouthguard and lose teeth that would not have been damaged had proper precaution been taken. It only takes a few seconds to put a mouthguard in and a fraction of a second to lose unprotected teeth.

7. Habitually sucking on lemons or limes will remove the enamel from your teeth and subject your teeth to bacterial decay.

8. Constantly keeping acid forming foods in your mouth most of the day is a very bad idea. Sucking on hard candy, eating cookies, cakes, and other high-carbohydrate snacks, keeps the acid at concentrated levels in your mouth, and dissolves tooth enamel. Bacteria utilize these massive quantities of sugary food to produce lactic acid and in turn this makes the acidic condition in your mouth even worse.

9. Consuming diet and carbonated beverages throughout the day keeps the acid level in you mouth at a PH level where teeth are demineralized.

10. Chewing regular or sugarless gum constantly keeps your mouth in an acidic state due to chemical additives, or sugar included in gum. Even supposedly healthy chewing gums that include Xylitol frequently contain additives that are acidic and offset the benefit of Xylitol.

11. Drinking canned and bottled fruit or vegetable juices throughout the day will keep your mouth in a highly acidic state and most of these products contain high amounts of added sugar content that feed bacteria in your mouth. Between the acid in the fruit drink and the lactic acid produced by the bacteria, the minerals will be dissolving from your teeth.

12. Sipping sugared coffee or tea all day will keep your mouth in an acidic state sufficient to begin dissolving tooth enamel. If you choose to drink cold brewed coffee without sugar and cream, the PH level can be kept safely just below neutral. Tea can be found that is low acid as long as you do not add cream and sugar.

13.   Ignoring cavities until your need fillings, crowns, or a bridge is another common error that leads to more traumatic problems. There is a price beyond money that you pay for dental repairs and we will find out why in the next chapter.

How Dental Procedures Impact Your Teeth and Your Health

It is with the best intention that we dutifully have our teeth cleaned, filled, crowned, bridged, and root canaled. The fact of the matter is that all of these dental procedures come with varying degrees of risk, most of which you will soon understand need to be avoided at all costs.

The least invasive, and most beneficial of dental procedures is the simple dental exam followed by a cleaning if plaque and tartar have accumulated on your teeth. Even having your teeth cleaned carries the risk of permanent gum damage if dental tools separate the gum line from your tooth, effectively creating a pocket where bacteria accumulate. Once bacterial colonies grow in a protected pocket below your gum line they are very difficult to control and remove.

It is my hope that as you read about the risks associated with more aggressive dental procedures, you will become highly motivated to take the actions necessary to avoid some of the life altering problems that often occur as you progress through the different levels of dental care at your dentist's office. The following information may forever change your perception about the benefits of dental work. Let's start by discussing dental fillings, the least dramatic repair to your teeth.

Fillings

Are your fillings slowly killing you? Well, they could be and there is plenty of scholarly research to back up the fact that some materials commonly used to fill teeth are extremely toxic. Among the heavy metals used in dentistry that are known to be toxic are mercury, silver, nickel, palladium, and copper. Heavy metals tend to accumulate in human bodies and, if not metabolized, can eventually reach a tipping point where poisoning symptoms begin to manifest.

The most common material used by dentists to fill cavities is silver amalgam, an alloy containing 50% or more mercury, and other metals such as silver, copper, and tin. Mercury just happens to be extremely toxic and can damage your kidneys, brain, and lungs. Mercury poisoning is linked to a wide range of disease symptoms. According to a 2007 abstract published at the National Center for Biotechnology Information website, vapor emitted from amalgam tooth fillings accounts for the most widespread exposure to mercury in humans.

The U.S. Food and Drug Administration depends on panels of experts for technical advice. Despite repeated advice from its own experts, the FDA has failed to follow its panel's advice to eliminate mercury from dental fillings for pregnant women and children. According to the FDA website (http://www.fda.gov/MedicalDevices/ProductsandMedicalProcedures/DentalProducts/DentalAmalgam/ucm171094.htm), "Dental amalgam contains elemental mercury. It releases low levels of mercury vapor that can be inhaled. High levels of mercury vapor exposure are associated with adverse effects in the brain and the kidneys." Still, the FDA considers exposure to mercury evaporation from fillings to be safe for pregnant women and young children.

Silver amalgam is presently banned in Denmark, Sweden, and Norway. On May 12, 2011 the Parliamentary Assembly Council of Europe, in a report to its members, (http://assembly.coe.int/Main.asp?link=/Documents/WorkingDocs/Doc11/EDOC12613.htm), advised its 47 member nations to restrict or prohibit the use of amalgam in dental fillings. Even though the American Dental Association and the FDA stick to their position that silver amalgam is harmless, you can demand other options.

If you already have a significant number of amalgam fillings, there is a chance that you may be experiencing symptoms of mercury poisoning. Research on monkeys revealed that mercury released from amalgam dental fillings into monkey tissues, (http://www.ncbi.nlm.nih.gov/pubmed/2227216), began accumulating in body organs and tissues in just a few weeks, indicating that mercury vapor is a serious health issue for people.

To be clear, there are no completely safe materials to serve as permanent tooth replacement. When you are forced into getting a filling, always insist on a less toxic alternative such as gold, or a nontoxic gold alloy, porcelain, composite resin, or glass ionomer cement. If your dentist refuses to comply with your wishes, or dismisses your concerns as trivial, it is time to shop for a new dentist. There are plenty of dentists who no longer use silver amalgam, or are willing to make alternatives available. Either call local dentists and ask if they will agree to not use silver amalgam, or search for a dentist using the International Academy of Oral Medicine and Toxicology website at http://iaomt.org.

A major drawback to having your teeth filled is that the filling commonly fails within 8 to 10 years, and often much sooner. Once the bond between the filling and your tooth is broken, bacteria take up residence in the protected crack and begin the process of decaying your teeth. The problems start getting worse with more complicated procedures such as crowns.

Crowns

You should make every effort possible to avoid having a dentist crown your teeth. Although there are times when there is no good alternative other than a crown, there are several reasons that crowns are a very bad idea. First, the existing tooth to be crowned is usually ground to a stub, effectively removing any possibility of an alternative treatment. Once the main structure of your tooth has been drilled away, the portion that is left is subject to a variety of problems, none of which are very desirable.

There is no such thing as an inexpensive crown for your tooth. It is highly unlikely that your dentist will tell you that most crowns will fail within a 5 to 15 year period, with the majority of crowns failing at the lower end of their life expectancy or sooner. When a crown fails, you will very frequently lose more of your underlying tooth structure.

Here are a few of the reasons a crown will fail:

1. All of the decayed tooth may not have been removed before the crown was mounted on the tooth stub.

2. The cement beneath a crown frequently breaks and allows the crown to leak; bacteria invade the resulting crevice and, safe from all efforts at cleaning, immediately go

about decaying the remainder of the tooth.

3. The weakened tooth stub beneath the crown is more easily fractured or broken than your healthy teeth.

4. Low quality crowns have a very short lifespan and tend to break.

5. Biting sticky or hard objects frequently break the crown's cement, or the crown itself. Even crunchy vegetables are capable of destroying a $1,000 crown.

Frequently, people have little choice but to get teeth crowned. Once your teeth have been crowned, the probability of those same teeth causing expensive new visits to your dentist within just a few years is extremely high. Unfortunately, the situation just gets worse.

After a crown has failed, enough damage may have been done where a post cannot be inserted to support a new crown and you will have to have that tooth pulled. Next, many people make the worst dental decision of their lives by agreeing to having a bridge installed. When a bridge is installed, the two healthy teeth on either side of the missing teeth are ground down for the bridge to be glued onto. Given the short lifespan of dental crowns, and the much higher probability for bridge failure, grinding down two good teeth to mount a bridge on is an exceptionally bad decision.

Far too many people have learned the hard way that a

bridge over one missing tooth can quickly become a bridge covering three or four missing teeth when the bridge destroys what used to be healthy teeth. If you add a new bridge every time the old one destroys its supporting teeth, one missing tooth can easily result in the loss of four to six otherwise healthy teeth in just a few years. The reason that a dental bridge is a high-risk proposition is that there is far more torque and stress on a bridge while chewing than there is on a single crown.

If you have missing teeth, the safest alternative is yet another poor choice: a partial denture. They usually do not fit or look as good as a bridge, but there are substantial long-term benefits. Opting for a partial denture avoids losing healthy adjacent teeth when your dentist drills them away to mount your bridge, and you avoid the risk of eventual bridge failure and the loss of teeth it was anchored to. You will also be able to thoroughly clean and disinfect a partial denture and the adjacent teeth. With a bridge, you will never be able to clean the surface area between the bridged teeth and that area becomes a permanent safe haven for bacteria and plaque build up.

When you have partially decayed or broken teeth, you should get the opinion of several dentists and find out whether or not building up and restoring the damaged teeth is possible. If all else fails, a crown may be necessary, just do not be surprised at the problems you will likely encounter after your teeth are crowned.

Another serious problem is that many dentists are

buying low quality discount crowns and bridges made in China and India. There have been reported cases of lead poisoning from the products imported from China and fecal bacteria has been found in the metal. If you do have a crown or bridge installed, insist that it be made from domestic sources.

Topping the chart for dental problems you want to avoid is the ubiquitous root canal. By the time your teeth to get to the root canal stage you have effectively put yourself at risk for a wide variety of health problems that extend well beyond your mouth.

Root Canals

Dentists perform literally millions of root canals each year. During a root canal procedure, the nerve and pulp are removed from the affected tooth and it is theoretically disinfected and sealed. Once a tooth has sufficient damage that a root canal is the last available treatment, you have entered a zone where there are few good choices. Some dental practitioners advocate the removal of a tooth once the pulp has become infected, however this only presents another layer of seriously bad choices.

There are many events that can trigger damage to your tooth's nerve and pulp. The most common is bacterial invasion through tooth decay, however trauma from impact to the face, cracked or chipped teeth, multiple dental procedures on the same tooth, and other problems can trigger a crisis. Before you agree to have a root canal procedure, keep in mind that once the nerve and pulp are removed, you have destroyed the living part of that tooth. If the nerve is inflamed, instead of infected, there is still a possibility that your dentist can perform what is called a direct pulp capping procedure. When successful, direct pulp capping allows the pulp to heal and the tooth will be able to function at a more normal basis.

Inside the pulp of your teeth, blood vessels and nerves

are actively circulating oxygen and nutrients to maintain tooth health. There is an active fluid pressure that transfers fluid from the pulp into the surrounding dentin and then through the enamel out into the mouth through hundreds of thousands of little tubules. When the circulatory system inside your tooth is destroyed, the natural ability of your tooth to keep itself healthy has been removed. Once the nerve and blood vessels are removed, the remaining tooth structure gradually becomes brittle and subject to fracture.

A tooth that has been compromised to a point where a root canal becomes necessary is a tooth that may be very difficult to disinfect. Cleaning out the pulp, using a disinfecting agent to kill microbes in the canal, and subsequent filling of the tooth, are frequently not successful because bacteria can remain trapped within tubules and, in the anaerobic environment, begin the process of decay again. With nerves having been removed from the tooth, you will not be aware that decay is in progress while toxins and bacteria are being released directly into your bloodstream. Unfortunately, your dentist has no way to be absolutely certain that disinfection of the canal has killed all the bacteria. Although a great many root canals are successful, a very large percentage do not turn out to be successful.

A reinfected root canal can release potent levels of bacteria directly into your bloodstream and potentially make you vulnerable to a variety of degenerative diseases such as cardiovascular disease, disorders of the immune system, kidney damage, neurological disease, cancer, and other significant chronic health problems. Even worse is that the infected area can go unnoticed for years and is practically immune to powerful antibiotics because there is no way to deliver an antibiotic inside a tooth where no blood is circulating.

Does this mean that you need to go and have your old root canals removed? Not at all, the presence of a chronic disease does not mean that it is caused by an old root canal, although it could be a factor. If you suspect that a root canal has failed, your best bet is to have your dentist X-ray the tooth to see if there is inflammation around the tooth. Although it is not absolutely guaranteed that the X-ray will reveal new infection, it is better than just having a tooth removed without being better informed. Failed root canals can, and often are, repaired successfully. Once you have removed a tooth the alternatives are not very good and include having a dental implant, bridge, or partial denture, all of which come with their own related problems.

Once a tooth is removed several bad things begin to happen. Teeth to either side slowly begin to drift to fill in the gap and this can cause problems with your bite, possibly leading to jaw misalignment and jaw joint problems. After a tooth has been removed, that area of the jawbone begins to dissolve and continues dissolving over a long period of time. The process of bone resorption is why many denture wearers eventually have great difficulty eating anything but soft food. Once you are restricted to only soft food, you will find your health will suffer accordingly because you will tend to not eat the range of foods you need to maintain good overall health.

Your very best solution is to prevent tooth decay in the first place, or if decay has already set up, get the cavity repaired as quickly as possible. Tooth extraction should be your absolute last recourse and should include taking advantage of root canal procedures where necessary to save the tooth. Although endodontic therapy leaves you with a dead tooth structure in your jaw, and leaves you open to subsequent bacterial infection, the higher risk associated with a root canal procedure is still preferable to the consequences of tooth extraction.

By now, you should have a good basis for understanding the impact your oral health has on your overall health, and why it is critical that you are diligent in protecting both. Next we will discuss the mechanical cleaning and sanitizing process to help keep your teeth in good health.

Caring For Your Teeth

If you are fortunate enough to not have any tooth decay, then preserving the healthy condition of your teeth needs to be a daily priority. When you have experienced tooth decay, or a toothache, you need to realize that this is your body's way of saying that something is wrong. By now you know that there are far-reaching health consequences to dental disease and tooth decay and you need to seriously listen to what your body is trying to tell you. Making a commitment to a consistent cleaning regimen is very important.

If you already have bleeding, infected gums, the next few chapters will be important in helping you with a plan for dental self-care that is easy, inexpensive, and designed to help get your infected gums back on the road to recovery. Following the cleaning and dietary advice offered in this book will help reduce the chances of serious infection ever occurring again.

Remember, you are engaged in a battle for your dental health that will never end. There is no one-time treatment, permanent solution, or cure for gum disease and cavities. By using this book you will have the tools necessary to take personal responsibility for your dental health. The next couple of chapters are for people who are experiencing bleeding gums or pain. If these conditions do not apply to you go ahead and skip to the Cleaning and Sanitizing chapter.

Treating Bleeding Gums and Aching Teeth

This chapter and the next focus on immediate steps you can take if you are dealing with bleeding gums or pain. Obviously, if you are in pain you want relief as soon as possible. You may not be able to see your dentist for several days, so you need to give priority to slowing down the problem causing the toothache in the first place. Unless you have a broken tooth, this means mounting a direct attack on the bacteria that are causing the problem.

WARNING - your results with this temporary remedy may be so effective that you decide not to go to the dentist. That is a mistake. You may have a cavity that needs to be filled, plaque below your gums that you will not be able to remove, or you could have more serious issues such as oral cancer that need immediate treatment. Make an appointment and see your dentist as soon as possible. Your dentist is not the enemy here and the longer you put off dealing with the problem the more likely a simple dental procedure will turn into a complicated, expensive visit later on.

Now, here is what you need to do three times daily until you see your dentist:

1. Supplies you will need: table salt or Epsom Salt, 3% Hydrogen Peroxide (the same stuff you buy at your local grocery or discount stores), baking soda (Arm & Hammer brand will do nicely), and dental floss. It is highly likely you may already have all of these around the house. Having a Water Pik or other mechanical irrigation device would be ideal, but if not, at least have a plastic eyedropper on hand (DO NOT use a glass eye dropper).

2. Use the dental floss for the first cleaning phase. The objective is to remove any food particles and built up sludge from between your teeth.

3. In two ounces of lukewarm water dissolve 2 teaspoons of salt and add one ounce of 3% Hydrogen Peroxide. This will dilute the Hydrogen Peroxide to a 1% solution. This mixture is a potent sterilizer and killer of bacteria.

4. Pour some baking soda into the palm of your hand. Dip your toothbrush into the salt/peroxide solution to moisten and then dip the toothbrush into the baking soda making sure it is well coated. Brush your teeth with this mixture by spending about thirty seconds on each quarter of your mouth. Take about two minutes to gently brush your teeth as thoroughly as possible. Rinse your mouth with lukewarm water and proceed with the next step.

5. Reload the toothbrush as above and give your tongue a good brushing. Again, rinse with fresh water. Your tongue

provides a wonderful motel for bacteria. It is time to start evicting them.

6. Instructions are listed below for using either a plastic eyedropper or an oral irrigator, such as Water Pik, to irrigate your gums (Please do not use a glass eye dropper inside your mouth).

NOTE: The objective for this step is to force some of this sanitizing solution below your gum line. This is nearly always where the main infection and source of pain originate.

a.) Plastic Eye Dropper Method - fill the eye dropper with your sterilizing solution and place it at the crevice between your teeth and your gum line. Begin squirting the solution beneath your gum line by moving the eyedropper along the edge of your gums, being very careful not to jab the tip into your gums.

Use enough force on the dropper to get the solution into the gum line. This will probably sting, but you are already hurting or bleeding, so let's bring the infection under control. Work the eyedropper all around the gum line where you are bleeding or have a toothache. Next, rinse your mouth for at least one minute with the remaining sterilizing solution, then rinse with freshwater and you are ready for the final step.

b.) Water Pik or other mechanical irrigation tool - fill your container with a solution composed of 2/3 salt water and 1/3 Hydrogen Peroxide. The salt may be either table salt or Epsom salt, but mix it one tablespoon of salt to eight-ounces of lukewarm water.

You may want to adjust the Water Pik pressure setting to a lower level than normal to minimize pain from the jet of water on the infected areas. Now, use your Water Pik to thoroughly work the sterilization solution into your gums by running the tip along the crack where your teeth and gums meet. Clean your entire gum line. Rinse for at least one minute with the remaining salt/peroxide solution you mixed (DO NOT swallow the salt/peroxide solution), then rinse with fresh water and you are ready for the final step.

The final step is simply getting to your dentist and getting the attention you need, otherwise, the problem will only continue to get worse. The steps you just completed will temporarily kill the surface bacteria and give you some relief. If you have a deep abscess this treatment may not help much and you seriously need assistance from your dentist. Bacteria embedded in hard plaque formations will not be affected by this treatment nor will the bacteria deep within a cavity. The only way to remove bacterial plaque below your gum line is to have your dentist physically remove the built up bacterial colonies. Otherwise, the problem will continue to get worse. The only way to remove bacteria in a cavity is to drill out the infected area.

If you have a broken tooth, you will want to take precautions to protect it and the rest of your mouth.

Temporary Tooth Repair

Broken teeth in your mouth pose a hazard, as do cavities with sharp edges. If possible, you should try to fashion a temporary filling to prevent damage to your tongue and inner mouth. Then see your dentist as soon as possible. Before you attempt to seal any broken tooth or cavity you should always make sure to first disinfect and sanitize the tooth to kill as many bacteria as possible.

If you will be able to see your dentist quickly, one solution is to purchase orthodontic wax and mold it around the problem tooth. Before you cover the tooth take time to brush, floss, and disinfect the tooth with a salt rinse or peroxide. Most drugstores, and pharmacy sections in retail stores will have orthodontic wax available.

When you are unable to see your dentist in a reasonably short time frame, you may need to buy a temporary filling kit in the pharmacy area of a local store. The kits are cheap and somewhat effective. Your dentist may not be too happy to see your self-administered dental work, but it is better than just leaving the tooth exposed.

A problem with the temporary filling kits is that the mixture is not easy to work with, so be sure to remove any of the material that sticks to your other teeth. When these types of mixtures harden they can be difficult to detach.

When all else fails, obtain sugar-free gum and chew it until soft enough to cover the tooth. Obviously, this is not a great solution, but it beats cutting yourself and allowing the damaged tooth to remain exposed.

Cleaning and Sanitizing Your Teeth

Presently there is no permanent cure, treatment, or vaccination against periodontal disease, including dental procedures, homeopathic treatment, dietary regimen, or other miracle treatment. Anyone who tries to sell you on the proposition that if you buy and use his or her program guaranteeing that you will never be at risk of gum disease and tooth decay is deceiving you. On the other hand, once plaque is removed from your teeth and gum line, you will be able to reduce the probability of gum disease and tooth decay to an extremely low probability if you follow a reasonable eating plan, keep most sugar out of your diet, keep your teeth clean, and your mouth sanitized. That only leaves the possibility of fractured or broken teeth getting infected and you can play a major role in prevention by being very careful that you only use your teeth for chewing food and rejecting anything that requires applying substantial pressure with your teeth.

Approximately eight out of every ten people in the United States have some degree of gum disease. In addition, the odds are good that people who presently do have healthy gums will fall victim to the ravages of gum disease even though they may brush and floss their teeth several times daily. Mostly this is due to not understanding the critical interaction of diet, acid, and sugar.

The objective of the following information is to teach you a simple, inexpensive, system of dental care that will dramatically reduce your chances of having tooth decay, gingivitis, or periodontal disease. You will learn to fight gum disease where it lives and is most vulnerable. You will wage war with the bacteria in your mouth, on your teeth, and below your gum line where brushing and flossing never venture. To insure that you understand the importance of the cleaning procedures let's briefly discuss the role of bacteria and the importance of effectively managing their populations.

Nearly everyone understands that bacteria accumulating on the surface of your teeth can eventually lead to tooth decay and gum disease. What is less understood is why you can brush and floss every day and still become a victim of periodontal disease.

With healthy gums there exists a very small gap between the tooth and the surrounding gum tissue. Usually regular brushing and flossing will scrub away plaque that is constantly formed by bacteria from the raw materials in your mouth. When the gap between your teeth and gum line deepens into a small pocket, bacteria can colonize and grow there in relative safety away from the brushing and flossing that take place above.

The pockets that form below your gum line may be caused by minor injuries incurred while flossing, brushing with bristles that are too stiff, eating, dental procedures, or inadvertently gouging a hole in your gum line with a toothpick. More frequently, the gap between your gums and a tooth is gradually forced open by the growth of plaque deposits and the build up of tartar.

Tartar, also known as calculus, is a build up of minerals above and below the gum line. Tartar below your gum line generally cannot be removed by flossing or brushing and is usually removed with a scaler by your dentist. Bacterial plaque on your teeth is typically not thick enough to see, and if you do not remove it the plaque formation will gradually harden into tartar.

As the bacteria colonize and reproduce in the protected areas below your gum line, infection will begin along with the onset of sensitive and bleeding gums. This stage is usually labeled as gingivitis.

When the disease advances you will progressively lose gum tissue and suffer bone loss. In the final stages your teeth will become loose, start shifting, and will eventually fall out in the midst of much infection and pain. At the end stage your overall health will very likely be severely compromised as a result of chronic infection in your gums.

Every day in the United States, dentists are seeing patients suffering horribly with disfiguring, and extremely painful advanced stages of gum disease that should never have been allowed to progress to that state. You do not have to join their ranks.

Dental offices are not inexpensive places to visit. X-rays, cleaning, fillings, crowns, bridgework, dental implants, gum surgery, and other procedures are very expensive. In addition, another factor that is rarely mentioned is that any medical procedure has its risks and side effects, and especially so with gum surgery.

A dental procedure as simple as cleaning the plaque and tartar from your teeth presents an opportunity to damage your gums and allow additional subsequent damage from invasive bacteria colonization. Engaging in an effective program of dental self-care is so important because it dramatically reduces the possibility of your teeth and gums being damaged unintentionally by your dentist when invasive cleaning procedures are necessary.

With the information provided in this section you will have the ability to dramatically reduce the costs of dental care and the risks associated with undergoing dental procedures. Best of all, the steps are simple, safe, and inexpensive.

The following steps to obtaining and maintaining good dental health will be explained in greater detail in the next few chapters:

- Plaque Removal and Scaling
- Brushing and Flossing
- Dental Irrigation
- Disinfecting Rinse

Plaque Removal and Scaling

If you just had your teeth cleaned by your dentist you can skip this chapter and move on to the information about brushing and flossing. This chapter is all about getting started on the right foot. That means removing plaque and tartar. Going to your dentist for a checkup to see if you have plaque accumulation is an excellent first step. If you do have plaque formation, a good dental cleaning is highly advisable and will put you on the road to maintaining good dental health.

I also realize that due to certain phobias, financial considerations, and distrust of medical practitioners, that some of you will not visit a dentist until there is no other alternative. Most people hate going to the dentist and the popular belief is that fear is the main reason for avoiding the dentist. The real reason so many people avoid the dentist office is simply an inability to pay for the procedures. This section of the book is written from the viewpoint that the steps provided in this chapter are a poor substitute for having your dentist professionally clean your teeth. Unfortunately, huge numbers of people do not have access to free dental clinics and have no means to pay for expensive dental care.

The self-treatment advocated in this book is not meant

to be a substitute for urgent dental care. This section of the book describes self-care treatment for people who are not experiencing symptoms that require the attention of a dentist. You will have to determine for yourself the current state of your dental health in order to decide how to proceed.

If you are experiencing severe pain, swollen and bleeding gums, and some of your teeth can be moved with your tongue or finger, then obviously you need to visit a dentist to begin treatment immediately, even if it requires finding a dentist who will work out a payment plan for you. Chronic pain is your body's way of telling you that you are in trouble and you need to seek appropriate medical care from a qualified medical practitioner.

When all else fails, and you refuse to go to a dentist, there are a few tools you will want to consider acquiring to help remove the housing structures for bacteria that have been deposited on your teeth. You will need a dental scaler and a small dental mirror; both can both be purchased for less than $10 at nearly any store that has a pharmacy section.

Additionally, purchasing an inexpensive battery operated tooth polisher is recommended and they typically cost less than $20. The cleaning agent for the polisher should be Pearl Drops Tooth Polish or a tooth whitening toothpaste. The last item you will need is a mouthwash solution you can easily make from salt in your kitchen cabinet, and 3% Hydrogen Peroxide.

4 Steps For Self-Cleaning and Scaling Your Teeth

The steps below are meant to help you remove built up plaque and tartar. Plaque can be invisible to the eye, but often manifests itself as yellow areas near your gums. Be extremely careful when using any dental tools around your gums.

1. Thoroughly brush and floss your teeth. Next, to kill as many bacteria as possible, swish for thirty seconds with undiluted 3% hydrogen peroxide, then rinse well with fresh water. Flossing is still an important step in removing plaque colonies where a brush cannot reach between teeth and in tight places where teeth meet.

2. Using the dental scaler, gently pull up and around each tooth starting at the gum line. Do not attempt to scale below your gums and risk serious injury to the soft tissue. Do not scrape cavities that have formed. If you have cavities you need to get those filled as soon as possible to prevent additional tooth loss.

3. Once you have descaled all your teeth, proceed to floss again, brush, and repeat the hydrogen peroxide swishing to sanitize and kill freshly exposed bacteria. Rinse well with fresh water.

4. Polish all your teeth with the battery-powered polisher while being very careful to work closely and gently into the gum line without pressing the polisher onto the gums. You do not want to injure your gums.

Work the polisher into the crevices between your teeth as thoroughly as possible. The polishing process should help remove additional plaque and tartar missed by the dental scaler. Rinse well, then swish with the hydrogen peroxide again, spit and rinse your mouth with fresh water.

At the end of this process your teeth should begin feeling smooth and slick. If there are still rough areas, use the dental scaler very gently to clean the area and then polish the tooth again with the electric polisher. It is important to note that you should never allow the scaler to dig into your tooth enamel, rather the scaler should be slid along the surface.

Now that your teeth are cleaned, swish for a minute with a solution made with a teaspoon of salt dissolved in 1/4 cup of lukewarm water as a final antiseptic rinse. Spit and rinse with fresh water.

At this point your teeth should have a glassy smooth feel like you would have after a dental hygienist has cleaned your teeth. If you follow the daily maintenance routine suggested in this book you will grow accustomed to how your teeth should feel, and you will be uncomfortable when you skip proper maintenance for a day or so.

You can spread the plaque removal and scaling process out over several sessions if necessary. Just be sure to clean all your teeth as soon as you can. The objective is to remove materials from your teeth where bacteria have begun building plaque colonies that eventually lead to decaying teeth.

Also, you should be aware that the bacteria in your mouth are necessary and actually play a role in keeping you healthy by attacking viruses, protozoa, and other undesirable bacteria. The problem arises when we do not manage their numbers through good sanitary practices including the brushing and flossing information we will discuss next.

Brushing and Flossing

This step and the next steps, dental irrigation, and disinfecting, will be your daily routine for maintaining a state of good dental health. The previous step was the initial cleaning to give you a good head start on beating tooth decay and gum disease. Now we will cover the daily routine for removing newly formed bacteria colonies, disinfecting your mouth and gums, and allowing your gums to begin the healing process.

Your daily dental cleaning routine will consist of four important steps that will help you maintain a high level of dental health:

1. First, you will want to floss, if not every day, then at least once every two or three days. There will not be a lot of material about flossing in this section. Study after study has proven that flossing can help reduce plaque and tarter. Flossing happens to be very effective at cleaning the tight places where your toothbrush cannot reach between your teeth. Just take a few minutes at the end of the day to run a little floss between your teeth.

2. Mechanical brushing twice a day is absolutely necessary. Many people believe that just brushing once is all that is needed, and that is a wrong approach. If you read the section about bacterial biofilm, you will understand that the

growth of plaque biofilm begins within minutes after you have cleaned your teeth. The longer the biofilm has to grow, the more likely that a hardened plaque spot will occur near your gum line, or in a crevice, that does not get dislodged when you brush again 24 hours later. By the time you brush your teeth the next day the plaque formation may have hardened sufficiently that it can only be removed by scraping with a dental scalar.

If you take the time to brush twice a day you keep destroying the immature plaque biofilm and make decay in cleaned areas nearly impossible. Your cleaning will be done with a regular toothbrush or an electric model such as Sonicare or Braun.

3. Proper disinfecting irrigation of the gums at least once a day.

4. Disinfecting Rinse.

Mechanical brushing on a regular basis will sweep away newly formed plaque. In those very tight places where your teeth either actually touch, or happen to be very close, bacteria can colonize into plaque formations and set off tooth decay. Flossing between your teeth helps to break up the plaque and that is why it is advisable to spend a little time working floss between your teeth.

The materials you will need to complete the mechanical brushing for step 2 are:

1. Baking soda

2. Salt - either table salt, Epsom salt, or sea salt

3. Soft or extra-soft tooth brushes

4. Interdental brushes. Usually they are very low priced and packages contain two to six brushes and are available at nearly all drug stores

5. A Sonic or Pulsonic toothbrush such as Sonicare or Braun. These toothbrushes are highly recommended, but if you do not have the funds then consider saving a little money back for a future purchase. These devices have heads that oscillate at very high frequencies, are very effective at disrupting plaque formations, and do an excellent job of cleaning critical areas where gums and teeth meet. If you cannot afford to purchase one of the appliances mentioned, make sure that you are using a soft bristle toothbrush.

You need to brush your tongue. No excuses. Your tongue has an immense carpet of crevices and nooks that provide a major breeding factory for bacteria in your mouth. If you want to have good dental health you need to clean your tongue as part of your daily brushing activity. All you really need is a soft bristle toothbrush and any kind of non-fluoride toothpaste. Scrub gently, rinse, and see if you still have a coating of material on your tongue. If your tongue does not look reasonably pink, continue gently brushing until you have removed most of the yellow or white layer of material built up on your tongue.

The next cleaning step is something that you have probably never done. Wash out your toothbrush and then very gently brush the areas inside your cheeks, under your tongue, the underneath side of your tongue, the gum and cheek area between your teeth, and the roof of your mouth. This helps disturb bacteria colonies that are attached to hidden areas you never touch when brushing and rinsing. Rinse your mouth thoroughly.

Now, we can move onto the actual brushing of your teeth. If you just had your teeth cleaned by a dentist, ignore the three paragraphs after this one, otherwise continue reading. During the first three days use the initial cleaning process described next to remove as much hidden plaque as you can. After the initial intense cleaning period, use a non-fluoridated, nonabrasive toothpaste or tooth powder. To begin the initial cleaning period, in a small cup, or glass, dissolve one-half teaspoon salt (table sale, Epsom salt, or sea salt) per ounce of water. The salt solution is extremely important because salt is a very potent bacteria killer.

When you first start a serious program of dental hygiene self-care, one of your objectives is going to be the removal of plaque and tartar. If you have not recently had a dentist clean your teeth, and you did not use a scaler to remove plaque, then for the first three or four days you will want to only use baking soda as your toothpaste. After that you will want to use nonabrasive toothpaste so you do not wear down the enamel on your teeth.

Contrary to popular myth, baking soda does not kill germs nor does it effectively operate as an antiseptic. There are two functions that baking soda serves quite well: First it is an excellent mild abrasive; secondly, it effectively neutralizes acid in the mouth.

Don't scrub your teeth using a lot of force, just brush with mild pressure and let the abrasive action of the baking soda work to remove additional layers of plaque and tartar you may have missed in the descaling step. Rinse well and spit out the baking soda and salt solution because, if swallowed, it is very high in sodium content and can have adverse effects for people suffering from hypertension.

It is very important that you spend an adequate period of time brushing your teeth. Brush in terms of having four sections to clean in your mouth. Concentrate on one section at a time and spend at least 30 to 45 seconds on each quadrant while you focus your attention on making certain that each individual tooth is being cleaned. The cleaning for each quadrant should first be directed toward cleaning the area where your teeth and gums meet and up the front and back of each tooth. When all your teeth have been brushed front and back, spend a minute focusing your brushing on the grinding surface where your teeth meet.

During the few days you are using the baking soda as a toothpaste you will want to coat the small interdental brushes with salt solution and baking soda, then brush gently between your teeth to help scrub away the plaque that your regular brushing will not reach and flossing may not have disturbed. Using the interdental brushes will definitely help disrupt new or accumulated plaque that flossing will miss.

For the first week you should try to brush at least three times daily. Later you should strive to brush twice daily. One of the most important times to brush thoroughly is before you go to bed at night. After you have cleaned your teeth in the evening, never eat any food, or drink anything other than water. Eating before you go to bed simply gives the bacteria in your mouth plenty of food to consume during the night. When you sleep, your saliva flow is at its lowest and if there is plenty of food available bacteria will build up a potent amount of lactic acid that surrounds your teeth all night. During the day you are actively eating, and drinking, and the secretion of saliva around your teeth and gums helps flush away and buffer acid.

There is an alternative method for brushing your teeth called blotting. Although I have not tried the technique myself, it is based on the work of a dentist, Dr. Joseph Phillips. The technique requires a special small "Blotting Brush" used without toothpaste by tapping vertically at a 45 degree angle on your teeth. This tapping is supposed to slip the bristles under your gum line and remove plaque. Some people claim that it is a very good technique.

The next extremely important step in your cleaning regimen is irrigating the gum line area. Brushing frequently does not remove bacteria accumulation where there is a small gap in between the gums and teeth.

Dental Irrigation

Once you have removed plaque and tarter by scaling and brushing, dental irrigation may be the single most effective ongoing activity in maintaining good dental health. Still, it must be used in conjunction with other regular dental self-care techniques.

Brushing your teeth is very important in that it serves to continually break up the inevitable plaque formations that occur within hours after you clean your teeth. Brushing your tongue breaks up the largest single bacterial breeding area in your mouth.

The odds are, even if you do not exhibit signs of gum disease, or have cavities forming, you very likely have some degree of gum disease that will eventually surface as sore and bleeding gums. Regular dental irrigation on a daily basis, especially before bedtime, is a major factor in reducing and eliminating infections beneath your gum line.

Do whatever you need to do to purchase a dental irrigation tool like Water Pik or Interplak. This purchase is one of the most important of all the dental tools and appliances available on the market. We have used both the Water Pik and Interplak devices and either one will get the job done effectively. Generally, the Water Pik will be more expensive, so if your budget cannot absorb the higher cost then the Interplak will do.

If you have to choose between an electronic toothbrush and a dental irrigator, choose the dental irrigator and just use a manual toothbrush in conjunction with pulling a scaler over your teeth every two or three days. The dental irrigator is important and when combined with an electronic tooth brush, you have a very effective set of tools to prevent tooth decay.

You will first want to concentrate on attacking bacterial infection below your gum line, and then continue with an antiseptic cleaning routine for your gums. We will start with killing the infection below your gum line.

You will need the following materials:

1. Salt - Epsom salt, table salt, or sea salt.

2. 3% Hydrogen Peroxide available at nearly any grocery or discount stores.

3. Water Pik or other mechanical dental irrigator including, if necessary, a plastic eyedropper.

To begin your attack on bacterial infection you will first fill the Water Pik reservoir with a salt solution of one heaping teaspoon of salt per 8 oz ounce of water, stirred and dissolved well. It is advisable to mix the solution beforehand and pour it into the Water Pik or Interplak so you do not damage the plastic container while trying to mix the solution inside the water reservoir. Leave about 1/2-inch of the container empty, then fill the remainder of the container with 3% Hydrogen Peroxide.

You now have a very effective disinfecting solution that is extremely tough on bacteria. The salt creates an imbalance in the water solution between the bacteria and its surrounding environment. Through osmosis, water is leached out of the bacteria until it can no longer maintain cellular integrity and dies. Peroxide is also a well known bacteria killer.

Use this mixture for the first five days. For your regular gum irrigation and disinfecting schedule you will then use plain salt water for two days and then on the third day add peroxide as instructed above. It is not recommended that you use peroxide every day because prolonged use may irritate your gums.

To begin killing bacteria below your gum line, set the power level on the Water Pik to 2 and begin directing the water pulses to your gum line at a forty-five degree angle. If you have already been using a Water Pik then you should use the settings you are accustomed to using. In any case, start at a power level that does not cause you any pain and gradually work up to higher power levels, but never use so much pressure that it hurts or stings. If pain occurs, back off the pressure because you do not want to damage your gums. If you do not have a mechanical dental irrigator, you may use a plastic eyedropper to squirt the solution along your gum line.

When you have completed the irrigation phase you need to rinse your machine. Rinse the water reservoir thoroughly and run a small amount of fresh water through the dental irrigator to remove salt residue. Leaving salt water inside the machine will corrode the parts and cause it to start leaking. Cleaning and flushing the machine this way will prolong its useful life.

If this is the first time you have used a dental irrigation device you will be amazed at what is flushed from your gums. It will become crystal clear why brushing and flossing do not effectively clean your teeth to a level that makes periodontal disease unlikely. People who have swollen, sore, or bleeding gums will notice a dramatic improvement in the health of their gums within two or three weeks after beginning a good cleaning regimen that includes using a mechanical dental irrigator.

One of the primary reasons that dental irrigation works so well is that it is physically impossible for brushing and flossing to reach all the hidden cracks and crevices in your mouth where bacteria congregate in mind-boggling numbers. Disinfecting liquids have no such limitations and as the sterilizing solution is forced below your gum line under pressure, the same fluids are flowing into the tight places between your teeth, the ridges on the roof of your mouth, and other hidden bacterial shelters that you would never think of cleaning.

The disinfecting rinse described in the next section will complete the last phase of your battle. You will still have bacteria in your mouth regardless of how often you clean. Our main goal is to manage and limit their growth so they cannot do serious damage.

Disinfecting Rinse

The final step for cleaning your mouth is as simple as it sounds. You will finish your daily cleaning regimen with a final disinfecting rinse. The default mouth rinse for most people is a commercial mouthwash. You really should not be using off-the-shelf mouthwash products because of toxic materials that can be, and are, absorbed directly into your body while in your mouth.

One example of the many toxic ingredients found in commercial mouthwash products is Benzoic acid. According to the ScienceLab.com Material Safety Data Sheet, "*The substance is toxic to lungs, the nervous system, mucous membranes. Repeated or prolonged exposure to the substance can produce target organs damage.*" The MSDS for another mouthwash ingredient PEG-40 says, "*Slightly hazardous in case of skin contact (irritant, permeator), of eye contact (irritant), of ingestion, of inhalation.*"

Usually, the toxic ingredients in commercial mouthwash products are not isolated. More typical is that all of the various toxic ingredients are all included together in the same product. Another example of toxicity for a common mouthwash ingredient, Poloxamer 407, comes from the NIH at http://www.ncbi.nlm.nih.gov/pubmed/17096184 which states in part, "*Poloxamer 407 has been held responsible for lipidic profile alteration and possible renal toxicity..."* yet each of these individual ingredients is considered to be safe in small doses. How safe can a dose of multiple toxins be when included in one bottle and consumed on a regular basis over a long period of time? I would rather leave the risk to more courageous people and stick with disinfecting solutions known to be less hazardous.

Here are some of the supplies you will need for your regular disinfecting schedule:

1. You should use your own salt solution rinse. Salt can be table salt, Epsom salt, or sea salt – mixed one or two teaspoons per 8 ounces of water.

2. 3% Hydrogen Peroxide – available at nearly every grocery and discount store.

Each day after brushing your teeth and irrigating your gums, you will want to do a final one-minute rinse by thoroughly swishing the salt solution. Spit, rinse with fresh water, and your teeth should feel as if a dental hygienist just finished cleaning your teeth. Every third day, swish a small amount of undiluted 3% Hydrogen Peroxide for thirty seconds, spit and rinse well. Do not ever swallow Hydrogen Peroxide or any of the other disinfecting solutions.

Now you have completed all the necessary cleaning steps to achieve good dental health. At least twice daily maintain a routine of flossing, brushing (including your tongue), dental irrigation, and disinfecting rinse. Remember that the very most important cleaning session is just before bedtime, so try to never skip your last cleaning of the day.

If you consistently follow these steps and recommendations you should achieve excellent results. Although the improvement in your dental health should amaze not only you, but your dentist as well, you would be wise to avoid pressure by your dentist to use any products containing fluoride.

The Fluoride Controversy

Well, it is time to wade into a bit of controversy about fluoride. Authorities on both sides of the fluoride debate cannot agree whether fluoride is wonderful or terrible for you, and each side presents compelling research statistics to support their position. Perhaps there is a logical explanation not taken into account that explains the discrepancies in research results presented by both sides. You may agree, or disagree with the conclusions presented later and that is your personal right, just be aware that you and your children will be directly impacted by your choices.

The holy grail of self-administered dental care in the toothpaste world, supported by most dentists and government agencies, is fluoride. Drink it, brush with it, smear it on your teeth; all things fluoride are supposed to be good for us. In the interest of doing the best for our children we provide them with the best fluoride toothpaste, fluoride mouthwash, dietary fluoride tablets, fluoride varnish painted on teeth, fluoride gel and foam rubbed on teeth, fluoride paste used by dentists to clean teeth, and of course plenty of fluoride fortified drinking water. As you read, keep in mind that children are also very prone to swallowing fluoride enhanced toothpaste, mouthwashes, and gels because of the sugary taste.

Governmental agencies, Dentists, Academicians, and independent researchers are deeply divided about the issue of fluoride. Some authorities present expert research proving that fluoride prevents tooth decay. Other authorities present very compelling evidence that the use of fluoride only gives the illusion of protection and eventually leads to a higher rate of tooth decay. A good resource where you can read detailed information about the opinions of parties on both sides of the fluoride issue is found at www.fluoridedebate.com, and you can also download the information as a PDF file.

Numerous scientific research studies have shown no difference in tooth decay between children who drink fluoridated water versus those who do not, and in some studies children drinking fluoridated water had more cavities than children drinking untreated water and receiving little additional supplemental fluoride treatment. On the other hand, there are educational groups and governmental agencies that hotly argue that overwhelming statistics prove that fluoride decreases tooth decay. An interesting experiment was conducted in Finland when, in 1992, water fluoridation was discontinued in the town of Kuopio due to local opposition to fluoridation. Of particular interest is the fact that between 1992 and 1995, with no water fluoridation, and a sharp decline in fluoride varnish and sealant applications by dentists, tooth decay actually declined. You may be interested in reading this interesting information at www.ncbi.nlm.nih.gov/pubmed/9758426.

One thing that is undeniable, other than the fact that

experts disagree about fluoride, is that among children and adolescents there is a quietly expanding epidemic of fluoride poisoning called Dental Fluorosis and the result is damage to permanent teeth. The CDC (Centers for Disease Control and Prevention) reported in the NCHS Data Brief Number 53, November 2010 that 41% of adolescents age 12-15 are experiencing Dental Fluorosis to some degree. The fluorosis trend is growing rapidly. You can read this information for yourself at http://www.cdc.gov/nchs/data/databriefs/db53.htm. Fluorosis damage causes wider tubule formation in the tooth's dentin, enamel layer pitting, and enamel pores to be exposed to bacterial invasion. In addition, fluorosis causes tooth enamel to become more brittle and easily fractured.

It does not take much of a leap in logic to realize that if fluoride is wreaking havoc on the growth of new teeth, it is at the same time impacting the growth of bones and vital organs. Also consider that about half of the fluoride entering your body is absorbed and accumulates in bones and tissues over your lifetime. The Fluoride Action Network (http://www.fluoridealert.org/fan-comments.html) submitted a document to the US Department of Health and Human Services reporting very interesting fluoride research including:

- Lower IQ in children exposed to high fluoride levels
- Brain damage in animal studies
- Skeletal fluorosis with conditions ranging from painful joints, osteoporosis or osteosclerosis, and a crippling stage where vertebrae are partially fused

- Disruption of the endocrine system
- A connection to cancer

In a letter to the Georgia Senate Majority Leader on March 29, 2011, former UN Ambassador Andrew Young expressed his strong interest in seeing Georgia's mandatory fluoridation law be repealed. Mr. Young expressed his deep concerns about the damage fluoride is having on teeth, tissue, and other bodily systems.

So, what is the big deal about fluoride anyway? Although there are many types of fluoride, the main two sources consumed by people are calcium fluoride and sodium fluoride. Learning a little information about the two primary forms of fluoride will be useful.

1. Calcium fluoride is a naturally occurring mineral known by the names fluorspar and fluorite, and is considered relatively harmless. The reason calcium fluoride is thought to be relatively safe is that two fluorite atoms bind to one calcium atom and become an insoluble compound. Most groundwater contains some calcium fluoride and, when ingested, only a small amount of fluoride is released into your bloodstream because it is bound to calcium. It is due to the very high concentration of calcium fluoride in the drinking water of certain towns in Colorado and Texas that water fluoridation became an accepted practice worldwide.

Around 1901, a Colorado dentist named Frederick McKay noticed brown stains and mottled spots on the teeth of many residents in Colorado Springs. In reports published in 1925 and 1928, McKay observed that low rates of tooth decay were associated with the stains and spots. The stains and spots that McKay noticed are also indicative of fluoride poisoning that results when the concentration of calcium fluoride is too high in water supplies. In 1931, the chief chemist at ALCOA provided McKay with evidence that fluoride was responsible for the unusual effect on teeth. Naturally, ALCOA was pleased with this favorable result and became the leading advocate for mandatory fluoridation of public water supplies since this presented the company an opportunity to make money selling sodium fluoride, their toxic waste byproduct produced from manufacturing aluminum. Interestingly, no serious early attempt to examine the difference between calcium fluoride and sodium fluoride seems to have ever been made.

    H. Trendley Dean, a dental surgeon with the US Public Health Service, confirmed McKay's research and determined that if the amount of fluoride in water could be kept at a level of 1 ppm, then the spots and stains would not appear on teeth, and tooth decay could be prevented. Fluoridation moved forward thanks to H. Trendley Dean's research, which is still considered the foundational basis proving the validity of adding fluoride to water, toothpaste, mouthwash, and other dental products. Unfortunately, governmental agencies have never amended their position on fluoridation even though in 1955, Dr. Dean was forced under oath to admit that his research data proving the benefits of fluoride was not valid (City of Oroville vs. Public Utilities Commission of the State of California, Oroville, California, Oroville, California, October 20-21, 1955.)

2. Sodium fluoride, and hexafluorosilicic acid (used in the production of aluminum) are the forms of fluoride added to municipal water supplies. Sodium fluoride has been used in products sold to kill roaches, water bugs, ants, silverfish, rodents, and as an ingredient in professional insecticide products; yet, it is considered safe enough to be included in toothpaste, mouthwash, and as a dietary supplement tablet for human consumption. Fluoride entering your body without an attached calcium atom will seek to bond with calcium in your tissues and bones, eventually leading to brittle bones as fluoride accumulates over a lifetime. MedScape.Com has an interesting set of articles about fluoride toxicity you can read at emedicine.medscape.com/article/814774-overview.

There is no question that based on available research, fluoride appears to stop tooth decay. On the other hand, there is no question that there are studies showing that fluorosis poisoning and tooth decay are higher in areas with water fluoridation than non-fluoridated municipalities. There has to be a common link that will explain how such disparate conclusions are reached. To narrow down what is the actual beneficial function of fluoride we can reference information provided in the July 2000 issue of The Journal of the American Dental Association (jada.ada.org/content/131/7/887.abstract), which indicates that the primary benefit from fluoride is derived from topical applications The abstract indicates that fluoride applied directly to teeth stops tooth demineralization that occurs from bacterial metabolic functions. If, according to the ADA, the primary benefit is application of fluoride directly to teeth, then what is the point of drinking a highly toxic substance?

According to Canadian dental research conferences in 1990 and 2001 (Research review - Fluoride 43(4)205–214 - October-December 2010), researchers found no clinically significant effect on bacteria from fluoride in toothpaste or mouthwash. In regard to the effect on bacteria from fluoride in drinking water the report stated, *"If high F concentrations, used directly on the teeth are unable to control microbial activity, it seems unlikely that the low F concentrations in fluoridated drinking water can limit microbial growth or metabolism in any clinically relevant manner."* Additionally, their report stated, *"In fact, no available research has shown that F at 1 ppm in water significantly alters plaque metabolism or plaque growth (bactericidal effects)."* The only other plausible explanation the researchers could reach is that oral bacteria have somehow become resistant to fluoride.

At this point I will offer a layman's opinion, based on the available research, about why fluoride appears to be effective at preventing tooth decay to some researchers, and not effective to other research groups. A likely answer is that concentrated fluoride can kill bacteria and inhibit bacterial growth since it is a potent toxin. In order for fluoride in drinking water to effectively prevent tooth decay, it will have to be consumed at levels sufficient to induce fluoride poisoning over an extended period of time, and this would seem to be confirmed by soaring rates of fluorosis in adolescents and children.

The high level of fluoride poisoning in children does not stop enamel erosion by bacterial and dietary acids, but it does allow pitted enamel to remineralize and incorporate fluoride ions into the calcium remineralization process. The result is harder enamel that is increasingly more resistant to acid erosion. This "strong teeth" side effect from excessive fluoride results in hard, brittle enamel that is easily broken, fractured, or chipped. Fractured enamel allows successful bacterial invasion where decay sets up safe from fluoride, brushing, and rinsing. Fragile, easily fractured teeth built with fluoride would account for why researchers have found a higher incidence of tooth decay in areas with fluoridation versus non-fluoridated towns. In areas with fluoridated water there is probably a lag time in tooth decay because of the initial toxic effect fluoride has on bacteria. Eventually the fluoride protected teeth become brittle, then fracture and break at a significantly higher rate than teeth built without fluoride. Bacteria invade the fractured teeth and tooth decay begins.

Keep in mind that the statements above are just my opinion, offered to make sense of conflicting results from reputable scientists. You may reach a different conclusion and it is just fine if we disagree. At this point, again my opinion, there is no compelling reason to ingest fluoride as it is a known toxin equally as deadly as arsenic, lead, or mercury. Dentists recognize that chronic fluoride poisoning is a risk for their patients, and if health professionals recognize the potential problem then it only makes sense to take precautions. There are better ways to keep your teeth healthy without resorting to drinking an industrial waste product, brushing with it, swallowing it in tablet form, or rubbing it on your teeth.

Sad to say, but if you want to avoid ingesting fluoride, there are not any inexpensive ways to remove fluorine from your drinking water. Choosing to drink distilled water from plastic bottles to avoid fluoride is problematic since the water will usually contain toxic chemicals that have leached out from the plastic. You certainly can avoid buying products containing fluoride and especially so for vulnerable children.

Most of the little water filters that attach to a faucet do not remove fluorine. There are a few counter top fluoride removing solutions that screw onto your water faucet and initially cost about $100, then $30 every three months for filter replacement. Also, there are larger, more expensive fluorine filtering counter top units that cost around $300 and hold a couple of gallons of filtered water ready to use. Then there are the reverse osmosis systems that cost $200 to $300 and produce relatively pure water, but come with plumbing costs and high maintenance expenses. Last, there are water distillers that turn water into steam and produce decent water. Home water distiller units are priced from $200 to $600.

It is your choice to consume and use fluoride based products, however you need to be prepared to accept the potential long-term consequences of that choice. Personally, I prefer to take a cautious approach and ingest as little fluorine as possible. There is too much conflicting evidence to convince me that fluorine actually has beneficial role to play in human health. Just a few of the preventative measures discussed next will go a long way toward protecting your dental health.

Preventative Measures

There are a great many things you can to safeguard your teeth and reduce the chance of tooth decay and gum disease to an absolute minimum. Of course, keep in mind that the greater the amount of dental work already in your mouth, the greater the probability you will have dental problems in the future. The reason for this is that fillings slowly work loose, crack, break, and are dissolved by acids in your mouth. The cement in crowns tends to fail very frequently, allowing bacteria to hide and grow safe from your cleaning efforts. Teeth that are relatively healthy, and have had a few minor fillings, present less opportunity for dental work to fail you. Below are a few things you can do to help keep your teeth in good shape.

1. Follow the cleaning and sanitizing regimen presented in this book twice a day.

2. When you eat, take a moment and run dental floss between your teeth to quickly remove food particles from between your teeth. Follow this by rinsing as described next.

3. After eating or drinking something acidic, you can dramatically offset the acid PH in your mouth by taking a moment to thoroughly rinse. When you are away from home take a little time to rinse your teeth with water. When you

are at home, or somewhere that you can keep a container of rinse solution, you will be able to quickly buffer the acid in your mouth by using a mixture of one teaspoon of baking soda and one teaspoon of sea salt mixed in a cup of water. At home you can keep any unused solution in your refrigerator unless your teeth are sensitive to cold, then just make a fresh batch of rinse solution each morning and keep in a sealed container. The Ph of sea salt is neutral and is very effective at killing bacteria, and baking soda neutralizes acid.

4. Brushing your teeth immediately after eating is a poor idea. The reason is that bacteria instantly begin feeding on the food you ingest and they secrete lactic acid. The acid from the bacteria, and any acidic food, immediately softens your tooth enamel and, depending on how acidic the food is that you consumed, it may take 30 to 60 minutes for your tooth enamel to harden sufficiently so you do not scrub it off with a toothbrush. It is particularly important that after eating or drinking acidic foods such as fruit, carbonated beverages, sweets, and other high acid items, that you wait at least an hour before brushing your teeth even if you rinse with a neutralizing solution.

Brushing your teeth before eating to remove as many bacteria as possible, then flossing and rinsing afterward is a much better practice for preserving your tooth enamel. Brushing and sanitizing before you eat dramatically reduces bacteria populations and this will result in a much lower level of lactic acid being produced by bacteria after you eat.

5. Eating a piece of hard cheese, or chewing celery right

after you eat will generate saliva to help bring the PH level in your mouth back up. An abstract published in the National Institutes of Health Library, http://www.ncbi.nlm.nih.gov/pubmed/7993600, revealed that patients undergoing cancer therapy consumed hard cheese for five minutes and experienced significant rehardening of tooth enamel. When you are away from home, and unable to brush or rinse, carrying a few pieces of hard cheese to consume after eating a snack or meal may be helpful in neutralizing the acid in your mouth and kick starting the enamel remineralization process.

6. One of the most critical times to clean and sanitize your mouth is just before bedtime. Once you have brushed and sanitized, do not eat anything and only drink plain water. At night, the saliva flow in your mouth reaches its lowest level and this creates a more acidic environment. Feeding the bacteria in your mouth before you go to bed allows their population to grow significantly and produce lactic acid. With reduced saliva flow at night the acids remain on your teeth and by morning will have softened and demineralized your teeth.

7. If you have silver amalgam fillings do not use hydrogen peroxide as a cleaner or mouthwash. Mercury is released from the amalgam by the corrosive bleaching effect of peroxide. Acidic foods and beverages accelerate the deterioration of amalgam fillings and dissolve the bond between your teeth and the filling. This allows bacterial invasion into crevices where subsequent tooth decay can begin. Strive to keep your mouth as PH neutral as possible

to preserve amalgam fillings.

8. Do yourself a favor and cease the consumption of carbonated diet and regular soft drinks, canned or bottled fruit juices, and sugar laden junk food. This will reduce the acid load in your mouth and improve your overall health.

9. The most important thing you can do for the health of your teeth and your body is to quit consuming sugar and sugar derivatives included in processed food. At the very least, only consume sugar with regular meals and no food or beverage containing sugar between meals. Keep in mind that there is a vast difference between the sugar in fresh fruit and the sugar in candy or soft drinks. As you have already learned, sugar suppresses the hormonal messages regulating the metabolic function of your teeth.

With determination, you can successfully preserve your teeth for a lifetime. Just don't get overwhelmed because as we discuss next, the secret to success lies in attention to the small things you can control.

The Golden Key To Success

There is a way of thinking and acting that leads inevitably to any destination, whether good or bad. It is easy to read and agree with the information in this book, take a few positive actions, then slip back into your old rut. Our habits are nearly always what lead to the present condition of our health.

To put a fine point on the matter, it is the little things in life that make all the difference. Let's compare the hypothetical lifestyle of two neighbors who are the same size and weight. Maybe you are the first person in our example. So, if you eat three cookies today and you are just too busy to exercise, you are not going to be noticeably heavier than you were yesterday. If you eat three cookies a day for the next month, you may gain a slight amount of weight, but probably not enough worth noticing. Eat three cookies a day for a year and you will wonder how you gained all those extra pounds.

On the other hand, each day your neighbor may do five minutes of squats, a couple of minutes of push ups, and only eat fruit for a treat. You may think that your neighbor does so little exercise that it is a joke because she will not weigh less tomorrow than she does today. At the end of a month there is really not much difference between her weight and yours so there is little to be disturbed about. Months pass and at the Christmas party you wear a baggy dress to cover up the new, larger you while your sleek, curvy neighbor is wearing a scandalous looking dress that looks like it was painted on, and worse, it looks damn good on her.

This is the way life actually works. The really big results in life, unless you accidentally hit a lottery, almost always come from a sustained series of small actions taken on a daily basis. If you consume a diet of commercially prepared foods every day because you just do not have time to prepare better meals, or you just do not know any better, you are not going to notice any difference in your health next week, next month, and probably not even next year. Twenty years of such eating and you will be a candidate for a variety of surgeries and multiple pharmaceutical drugs for conditions including depression, diabetes, heart disease, cancer, and other degenerative health problems. The destruction of your health is a very large price to pay for convenience food.

For a great many people, the first warning sign their body gives that all is not proceeding well is when a little tooth decay begins bothering them. Next are fillings, crowns, then dentures, all accompanied by a wide variety of mystifying aliments, fatigue, and depression. Few people seem to understand that those aches and pains are nature's way of letting you know that you need to change what you are doing because there are sound dietary reasons for the negative changes you are experiencing.

As you learned earlier in this book, what you put into your mouth can bring the circulatory system in your teeth to a dead halt. Instead of bringing nutrients to the living tooth structure and cycling waste back out, the process is stopped. When this natural metabolic process is brought to a halt in your teeth, what else do you think may be happening to your body that you do not know about? Do you think that there is at least a remote possibility that additives in your food, that only a chemist can decipher, are causing silent malfunctions in your body's critical processes? Sure, you may not notice any effect today, tomorrow, next month, or next year, but what about the consequence of consuming dozens of different toxic chemicals every day for years? Might that have an impact on your health?

Wherever you are in life, you can begin making small positive changes. You probably will not see any significant health improvement tomorrow, next week, or next month. Try a year of better dietary and oral hygiene habits and see if the change isn't dramatic. Making small choices every day not to consume sugar and chemicals will, over a period of time, have a major positive impact on your teeth and your overall health. Choosing to clean and sanitize your teeth twice a day will result in healthier teeth compared to a few years from now if you only clean when you have the time, if at all.

Small choices and small actions every day lead to big outcomes, and so does failing to choose and act wisely. In the end, your dental and physical health is pretty much in your hands and is determined by your personal daily decisions. The only things your dentist can really do for you are drill and fill the bad decisions you made for your teeth. Your physician can medicate and operate on you at the tail end of a long series of poor dietary choices you have made. It is up to you to choose wisely, frequently, and consistently.

You have probably heard enough by now, so it is time to wrap up this book. I just have a few final thoughts to pass on to you in the next chapter.

Summary and Conclusion

Assuming that you read this book without skipping chapters, you have built a foundation of knowledge on which to base rational decisions regarding your dental and physical health. Often, the difference between something sounding like a good idea, and having a compelling reason to make a commitment you stick with, is to understand the underlying reasons for the actions that you take. I hope that I have transmitted enough information in this book for you to make choices based on the knowledge that there are specific reasons for actions will benefit you now and in the years to come.

Ideally, your family and friends will participate by taking advantage of your knowledge. In the end, each individual is responsible for their actions and has to live with the consequences of their own choices. You may not be able to convince your spouse, children, relatives, or friends that their constant dietary intake of sugar is lethal to their dental health. The best you can do is set an example for others to follow with the understanding that they may never change their habits. Too many people reason that if they are not having a problem with health now, then they will worry about it when and if the time comes.

The ideas presented in this book are relatively simple

and easy when you seriously consider the benefits. Here is a quick rundown of what we have covered:

- You know why sugar stops the natural metabolic function in your teeth.
- You understand the role that acid plays in destroying your teeth.
- You know that a cleaner diet plays a major role in your dental and physical health. In particular, the presence of vitamin D3 and other fat soluble vitamins are of exceptional importance.
- You can appreciate the reasons why the more dental work in your mouth, the more difficult and expensive it will be to maintain your dental health. The less dental work installed in your mouth the better off you will be in all respects. All reasons for consistent actions that lead to long-term desirable results.
- You now have a solid plan for cleaning and sanitizing your teeth to insure good dental health.

At this point you have the information and means to effectively manage your dental health. I know from my own personal first-hand experience, and the experience of my husband, and friends who have implemented these self-care methods, that the techniques are very effective.

It took me a long time to realize that the dental and medical professions are primarily focused on treating the symptoms, and not the causes of dental and medical problems. This is not meant to criticize those professions because they do provide a fundamental service and play a vital role in our society. Information is available for people to make wise decisions about their health. The biggest problem for too many people is that making the right choices is just too inconvenient.

Perhaps future advances in dentistry will make tooth decay and gum disease a thing of the past. Technologies being tested that show promise, but are not publicly available, include a couple of interesting advances. Research indicates that glucansucrase enzyme may be effective at stopping bacteria from adhering to tooth enamel. This enzyme could be easily delivered in toothpaste or food. Another interesting development is research conducted with a peptide based fluid known as P 11-4. When the peptide fluid is inserted into a cavity, it seeps into the damaged micro-pores and forms a structure that attracts calcium from saliva to regenerate the tooth from within.

Other technology under research includes a vaccination that would supposedly make you immune to dental disease. Unfortunately, this may be a potential health disaster waiting to happen. Genetically modifying organisms to combat other living organisms is subject to causing bacterial and viral mutations that are worse than the original organism. An example of this is the quiet crisis going on with failing genetically modified crops where normal crop pests have adapted into super bugs.

Your dental and physical health are your personal responsibility, not that of your medical provider. It is up to you to maintain the conditions necessary for your body to function properly. Dentists and doctors do an excellent job performing the procedures they have been trained to do, but their training rarely includes teaching you to follow a holistic approach designed for prevention. That is where you have to enter the picture and take action by doing the things that will insure that you rarely have to visit a dentist.

Best wishes and good health.
Alicia Smith

Printed in Great Britain
by Amazon